Healing Power of
Meditation

Dr N.K. Srinivasan

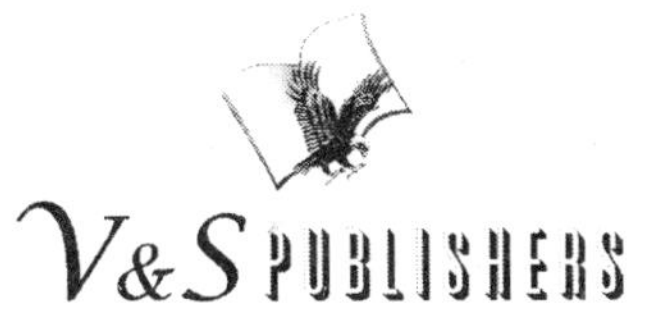

Published by:

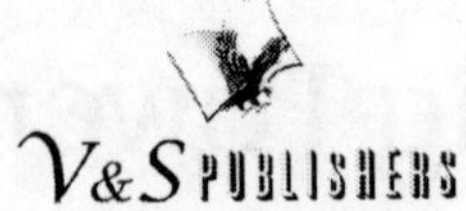

F-2/16, Ansari Road, Daryaganj, New Delhi-110002
☎ 011-23240026, 011-23240027 • *Fax:* 011-23240028
Email: info@vspublishers.com • *Website:* www.vspublishers.com

Branch : Hyderabad
5-1-707/1, Brij Bhawan (Beside Central Bank of India Lane)
Bank Street, Koti, Hyderabad - 500 095
☎ 040-24737290
E-mail: vspublishershyd@gmail.com

Branch Office : Mumbai
Jaywant Industrial Estate, 2nd Floor–222, Tardeo Road
Opposite Sobo Central Mall, Mumbai – 400 034
☎ 022-23510736
E-mail: vspublishersmum@gmail.com

Follow us on:  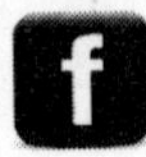 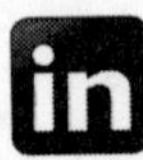

All books available at **www.vspublishers.com**

ISBN 978-93-813846-3-3

Edition 2017

Previously Published under the Name :
Safe & Simple Steps to Fruitful Meditation

Printed at : Param Offsetters, Okhla, New Delhi-110020

Om Sai Ram

This book is dedicated to

MY LORD SHIRDI SAINATH

Contents

Contents

Preface

This small book is aimed at providing practical techniques of meditation for the general reader. Whether religious or not, one can practise meditation for mind control to achieve mental poise (balance) and mental peace. In the modern, high-tension lifestyle, meditation for even 10 or 15 minutes can bring about great mental and physical relief and solace to a troubled mind. There are, of course, those who wish to pursue meditation as a spiritual effort or 'sadhana'.

We present several techniques commonly practised from Indian traditions over the ages. Starting with simple breath-watch, many methods used by yogis and monks are given in simple, easy steps, with numbered practice sessions. One should follow the steps carefully to derive maximum benefit. Certain meditations for healing are also included.

The present book carefully examines some of the controversial issues and presents the best approach or thinking known to the author. Several warnings are given so that the reader is not misled by teachers/gurus who profess wrong or misguided teachings or practice.

Since meditations advanced by Buddhist monks are very important, a chapter is devoted for such practices. In fact, these methods originated in India and later spread to China, Japan and Tibet under the care of Buddhist clergy. A detailed account of chakras and related meditations are given; this is one of the major topics, often misinterpreted in yoga literature. For a beginner, the chapters on the benefits of meditation and frequently asked questions (FAQs) would clarify many common doubts and help to strengthen one's interest in meditation.

It is hoped that this small book will enable a beginner to learn the basics and to practise meditation in easy ways. The practise of meditation, even in a small way, will gradually enable the reader to realise his or her full potential as a human on this earth. Perseverance is required.

27 July 2004

—Dr N.K. Srinivasan
Bangalore

1. Introduction

Meditation is a process that anyone can learn and practise. If you happen to be religiously inclined, certain types of meditations would appeal to you. If you are not, there are other types of secular meditations that you can practise.

In a sense, meditation is a natural process – as natural as your breathing. No one taught you how to breathe when you were born. Likewise, we all meditate, often unconsciously. When you are at the altar or pooja room at the home or in a temple or church or mosque, a few moments of thoughtless awareness may be experienced. But such moments are rare and fleeting, and may not make an impression in your mind. Here we are talking about *conscious meditation through practise,* with definite objectives.

The effects or results are bound to be long-lasting and under your control. You are aware of yourself as a meditator in the early stages, though at later times, you lose your awareness. Only when you come out of the meditative state, you feel: "My God, I was in deep meditation for nearly an hour."

Furthermore, the effects of meditation will be felt even after the formal meditative state is over... say for the whole day or for a few days. Meditative experience is similar to deep, dreamless sleep (*sushupti*) but with this difference – you are conscious of yourself in meditation but not so in deep sleep.

While meditation per se is a natural process, you need some kind of training and guidance to achieve effective results. A child may learn swimming very fast with little coaching.

A grown-up man or woman needs effective coaching to learn to swim – due to fear, stiffness of the body and lack of coordination. Likewise, a small boy with less cares and anxieties may learn meditation very fast, but for grown-ups, especially for an anxiety-ridden businessman or woman or a busy professional, unwinding first from tensions and then practising meditation are not easy skills. He or she needs training from an experienced master.

What would you learn from this book? There are yogis and seers who are constantly in a meditative state called *Sahaja Samadhi* – but everyone does not attain this state. Some go into trance for several hours – again a state reached by advanced yogis. While these states are not impossible for anyone, they are not easy to achieve either. What we explain in this book are more modest efforts suited to modern men and women – hurrying through life, with a burden of anxieties and worries – not for those who retire into retreats or the caves of Himalayas for months at a stretch. The practices are simple and easy to follow and can be practised for a few minutes to an hour or more each day.

Self-help Vs. Guru Teaching

A Guru or preceptor who can initiate you and monitor your progress is desirable. A *guru* literally means *'one who dispels darkness or ignorance'*. (The word "ignorance" has deep meaning in Hindu philosophy or Vedanta and we would not digress into that!)

But real, accomplished gurus are rare and may not be accessible to you... There are many gurus and teachers with very elementary knowledge obtained after a short course under a guru or teacher who proclaim their powers and begin to teach without much practice or experience (*'anubhava'*) on their own part. Then there are gurus attached to certain groups or organisations who teach, in a mechanical way, certain steps or methods with very limited understanding or appreciation of the deeper meanings of the processes. In fact, such gurus are aplenty in any large city and they even regularly advertise in the Yellow Pages or newspapers!

It should be added that there are great gurus in India, but they are not easily accessible for a variety of reasons. Some are totally unapproachable and would drive away any intruder disturbing their solemn penance. Some may give cryptic guidance through a chance encounter, if you are destined to receive their instruction and grace. For many young people, the rigorous lifestyle of some ashrams and yogadhams (yoga centres) are totally uncomfortable. (For many westerners or western-styled Indians, these ashrams or gurus are 'unliveable', as some would put it – except for a few students of philosophy or religion, who do their thesis work for a Ph.D. and somehow put up with these difficulties for a few months to complete their 'field work'.)

In this situation, one has to proceed via self-help possibilities with a book like the present one. This can be supplemented by short discussions with accomplished yogis, if possible. Further, study groups of like-minded persons called *'sat-sangha'* or retreats may do some good. If one can meet saintly persons, called *'sadhu sangha'*, it would be preferable. In this modern age, one can communicate through the Internet with a few reasonable teachers and masters to some extent. All these approaches are alternatives to guru teaching and can serve only as preliminary preparation.

As Hindu scriptures say, "If you are ready, a guru will seek you" or "If you walk one step towards God, He will run ten steps towards you". These sayings indicate the possibilities of divine intervention in your spiritual progress. According to Hindu doctrine, whether this will happen in this life or in some future birth is left to your destiny. One thing is possible... You can take the first step: "All journeys begin with a single step."

What is Meditation?

While there are several definitions of meditation, a simple and direct one is as follows:

Meditation is consciously directing your attention or thought to alter your state of consciousness... (In this process, you may reach a state of thoughtlessness or mind absorption.)

What is the Purpose of Meditation?

In other words, why would you like to meditate in the first place? For many, meditation may appear to be a sheer waste of time. Some are afraid that during meditation, their dark feelings and thoughts will surface, leading to depression and feelings of hopelessness.

Meditation, at the simplest level, is known to reduce your physical and mental tensions. The physiological effects such as reduction in blood pressure, metabolic rate, and alpha waves rhythm have been studied in detail and are well documented. Many meditators experience reduced tension and mental calmness even after short practise of meditation.

At higher levels of meditation, one can expect an understanding of a wider and broader view of life, more tolerance and expanding love towards all – slowly you leave anger and resentment behind. You become more forgiving and thereby capable of expanding zones of LOVE towards all – including your sworn enemies. This stage may be reached after a few months or after a year or so of practice.

At a still higher and advanced level of meditational practice, one would begin to perceive better and greater intuitive powers. (At the mundane, worldly level, this may help managers towards better decision-making.) Intuitive powers lead to inner guidance, particularly when one wants to make major decisions in life. Inner guidance will be received in abundance by any serious meditator. (See section on *The Benefits of Meditation*.)

At still higher levels, one can acquire psychic or occult powers and, above all, an ability to read others' minds and influence them. Such powers are derived without effort but, at the same time, should not be pursued for cheap thrills or for vain display or for making money.

For many, however, meditation is of direct interest towards healing of body and mind. Many diseases are of psychosomatic nature and would respond to meditational practices. Healing with meditation on chakras or nerve centres is a special technique. In this book, we briefly discuss this technique, though one may follow this instruction with specific guidance from a master.

The ultimate aim of meditation is, of course, spiritual development leading to liberation from the cycle of birth and death – Moksha or Nirvana or Enlightenment. This level can be reached after considerable practice with the grace of God or the Supreme Power. No one can say when and how this state will be reached.

The word *'Dhyana'* is used to denote meditation. Dhyana is one of the eight parts of the Eight-part or Eight-limbed Yoga, defined by the Sage Patanjali, called *Ashta-anga Yoga*. The eight parts are: *yama, niyama, asana, pranayama, pratyahara, dharana, dhyana* and *samadhi*. We shall discuss these steps in various sections. Patanjali's *Yoga Sutras* is the basic text for this yoga, which forms the main basis for Raja Yoga ('The royal yoga' or Yoga of Meditation).

Our aim in this book is to provide simple, practical procedures for various types of meditation with the necessary theoretical, conceptual background.

2. Conscious Listening

One of the first steps in meditation is to accept oneself and to love oneself. Listen to yourself. Accept yourself with all your defects, blemishes, shortcomings, limitations and past sinful deeds – do not use self-pity or criticise yourself. Having done that, ask yourself what good you can do in this world – tell yourself how you would love others.

Self-love is not an obsessive, narcissistic form of love, but only accepting your faults and weaknesses as real human weaknesses and focusing on how you would become better – this is possible only if you love yourself as a highly evolved human on this planet, who can consciously change at this time.

With this, you love others who also have their faults and weaknesses like you. Now spread your 'Wings of Love' to all. This also means that you forgive others, even your worst enemies, their bad deeds and things they have said about you or done to you. It is almost impossible to love another person without forgiving him. Harbour no hatred towards anyone.

Active listening to other people is the first step in loving others. Avoid hasty or instant judgements. Listen to others without judgement or criticism, absorb the other person's message; then you can review and criticise in your own mind what he or she has said.

We all experience fears of various kinds – fear of pain, injury and death. It is extremely difficult to overcome many types of fears. With deep meditation, our inner strength increases and we can learn to overcome fears. As all of us know, fears lead to anxiety and physical illnesses.

One of the fears is that of abandonment or loneliness. This fear arises in childhood and may persist much later. Many elders have this fear of being abandoned by their kith and kin. Here again meditation can help to overcome such fears, as you depend more and more on the Supreme Force or God to protect you, give you company and remove loneliness. Fear of death or loss of mobility afflicts one as age advances. Besides counselling, meditation helps to achieve mental poise and accept the inevitability of problems of advancing years and the ultimate end.

3. Love Heals

The greatest healing force in this world is LOVE. Love is an overused word that has lost much meaning in our modern world. The reason is that we do not have the capacity to listen to, to appreciate and to forgive others... We all understand the love of a mother for her child, called *'vatsalya'* in Hindu philosophy. There are other forms of love – there is a kind of love between a master and his servant. There is another kind of love between a woman and her husband. All these can be translated as love at higher levels – between the person and the Cosmic Beloved or the Supreme Force... While these are elaborated in Bhakti Yoga (the path of devotion), one should proceed with the steps given in the previous section to open one's heart towards others.

Practice 1

A simple meditational practice is as follows:

- Stretch your arms and keep your palms open towards the front, as you would do in blessing a person. (This is called 'Abhaya Mudra' in literature. *Mudras* are *signs* or *gestures* used in Yoga.)
- Say aloud three times: "I love all beings living on this planet."
- Visualise love radiating outwards from your heart towards all beings.

> **Note:** *This practice may appear highly imaginative. It is important to understand and follow the steps given in the previous section to appreciate and actualise this practice.*

Self-discipline

Before we proceed to describe the various meditation practices, we have to stress a few points regarding self-discipline. Serious students and followers of meditation must observe their own self-imposed rules of practices and social behaviour, such as:

1. Stick to a particular time and place for meditation. Be regular in practice. Even if you practise only for 5 minutes everyday, regularity will carry you forward, instead of irregular practise at odd times and in odd places. Create your own environment for meditation. You should not miss meditating even for a single day, except in case of emergency or serious illness.
2. Avoid the company of those whose talk is frivolous, scandalous, time wasting and trivial. You can keep your mind calm and serene if you follow this restriction. This also applies to watching meaningless programmes on TV and engaging in long conversations over the phone. Avoid wasting your energy by reading useless information in newspapers and magazines.
3. Associate with serious meditators and yoga groups or form your own group (*sat-sangha*).
4. Practise silence as much as possible; talk less and listen to good lectures or audio/video tapes. (You can practise total silence one day in a week.)
5. Observe other serious meditators closely. The company of saintly persons is one of the easiest paths for spiritual progress, called '*sadhu sangha*' in Hindu literature.

6. You may seek quiet spots and meditate for 10 to 30 minutes – for instance, on a lonely beach, in a quiet temple or church, a calm wooded park, etc.
7. Keep a journal or diary of your daily experiences. Note down even small or what appear to be trivial experiences or observations. You can show parts of your diary to others or discuss it with them; but for the most part, it is for your own analysis. Record both pleasant and unpleasant experiences. Review and record any definite progress once a month. (Note even small things such as getting angry with a stranger or intruder, showing impatience at a crowded place or in a long queue.)
8. Decorate the meditation room with pictures of saints and sages, and your favourite gods; avoid gaudy or bright cloth or drapes; burn incense if you wish; avoid keeping mundane pictures of scenery or tourist spots.

4. Meditation Techniques

Setting the Scene

One must first set the scene for peaceful and deep meditation. A few pointers:

- ✦ Keep your body comfortable with loose clothing;
- ✦ You should not be hungry or on a full stomach.
- ✦ Avoid meditation after a heavy meal; at least an hour must pass by after a heavy meal.
- ✦ Learn to sit still, without the hands fidgeting, legs shaking or simply moving about and the fingers twiddling something. Practise this!
- ✦ Keep the surroundings or the room cool, without draft or heavy winds; the room should be well ventilated. In India, being hot in most places, the best place is often a shady area under a large tree.
- ✦ Switch off the telephone, radio or TV. When you are in deep meditation, even the ticking of a nearby clock can be distracting for some persons.
- ✦ Keep the mind calm and not agitated or worried. (In your own mind, resolve any bothersome matter or situation before you sit for meditation.) Leave worries at the doorstep, as you leave your slippers.
- ✦ *Do not expect strange or unusual experiences – be your normal, usual self.*
- ✦ A positive step is as follows: recall moments of peace and serenity; visualise with closed eyes, places of calm you have visited before: a lonely beach, a quiet temple

or church, a fragrant garden with bright sunshine, a view of snow-clad mountains on a bright day, birds chirping in a cool garden, etc.

- **Maintain your mental stillness and tranquillity – even a few minutes will help.**

When to Meditate?

While one can meditate even at odd moments, for instance, while travelling in a bus or a suburban train, a serious meditator must allot a time for regular practice. Even if one meditates for only 5 or 10 minutes, if he does that at a fixed time everyday, the habit becomes more effective.

Early morning time is the best – soon after awaking. The body is well rested and the mind is calm at that time. Hindu sages recommend a meditation session between 4 and 5.30 AM, *called Brahma muhurtha,* suited for this practice. Hindu philosophers consider this time auspicious and sacred.

Another period suited for meditation is at night, before retiring to bed. You may feel tired, but you know the day's work is over and will feel mentally relieved. Before meditation, you can have some fruit juice or milk and a light walk for 5 to 10 minutes to refresh yourself. After that, you can sit for meditation. Hopefully, you won't fall asleep at that time!

There are yogis who meditate four times a day – early morning, noontime, at dusk and at night. Dusk period meditation is considered very effective, as the day changes into night, and there is a sense of transition and calmness when birds return to their nests and a certain quietness is felt, especially in rural areas. These four periods relate to *sandhya kalas* used by the pious for their *vandanas* or prayers. (*Sandhya* is a period of transition from night to daybreak, forenoon to afternoon and so on.)

Most people prefer to meditate twice a day, in the early morning and either in the evening or at nighttime.

Whatever be the time, establish a regular time for the practice. Regular practice is more important than the duration of meditation.

How Long to Meditate?

The initial stages of practice can be for only 5 to 10 minutes in each session. It is amazing how much you can progress even with such a short session. Gradually increase the duration to 20 to 30 minutes per session. It is important to continue meditation without any break. Therefore, don't keep looking at the watch every few minutes. Forget the watch. Forget the passage of time.

Certain gurus recommend only 20 minutes. But after some practise, you may be able to meditate even for an hour in a single sitting. If you reach that stage, you are indeed an experienced meditator by then. Note that you will experience extreme calmness or a blissful feeling only if you meditate for more than an hour or so. Some yogis, including the present author, meditate for more than an hour in each session.

You must adopt some methods of time management for this to happen. Even yogis and gurus are busy persons nowadays with several 'engagements'. It is important to tell others that you will not be available during the period of meditation and that you should not be disturbed on any account. Switch off the phone and alarm clock. Your family members at home should not disturb you.

Most meditators meditate in an isolated room or porch and put up a board, "Don't Disturb". It is important that no one touch you during meditation. You may experience a sensation like a severe electric shock if someone touches you. The author has experienced such shocks and even moments of convulsion when someone inadvertently touched him or called him aloud during meditation.

In the first few minutes of meditation you may experience a slow release of tension in the body and gradual control of the breath. Real meditation begins only after that stage.

Place and Posture

The place should be calm and without distractions at least in the early stages. Great yogis can meditate with their eyes open even in a marketplace or a noisy Indian bazaar. But the beginner cannot do that.

You should have a well-ventilated, warm room, which is often the pooja room in Indian households. Please avoid meditating in the bedroom or the common visiting room where the atmosphere is not conducive. There should be no cold draught or sunshine falling directly into the room to cause glare.

You should have a few pictures of your favourite God (Ishta Devata or Kula Devata – the god of your clan) or guru or favourite saints. In the Hindu household altar, one may find even 20 pictures due to various associations, as well as the pictures of presiding deities of famous temples in India. The room may be dimly lit. You can keep incense sticks and an oil lamp or burn candles, as you wish. Most Indians love to decorate the images and pictures with fresh flowers. (Avoid using plastic flowers since they give the feeling of artificiality.) Some may keep stone or metal images, according to their liking.

There are no rigid rules for the decoration of your meditation room. As time passes, you may be inclined to make changes in this room. Note the changes you want to make in your journal. Think about the plausible reasons for making the changes. Are they signs of your spiritual progress or changes in your attitude towards meditation?

The seat for meditation once received much attention. One should have a warm seat to sit upon for long periods during meditation. Yogis of the past used tiger skin or deerskin on a bed of grass. In the *Bhagavad Gita*, Lord Krishna gives details as follows: *Spread kusa grass (a bed of dried grass), and over that a layer of animal skin. The height of the seat from the ground must not be too low or too high.*

While this had much relevance in Vedic times, we can simplify the seat. Unfortunately, even today, some yogis use deerskin or tiger skin for display of their status as pontiffs. It is important that the seat is firm, not soft and warm. In modern times, a few layers of woollen rugs will do. Some may have a layer of pure silk – all these act as thermal insulators and may store electric (static) charge. In humble abodes of yogis, one finds mats made of straw, normally used in Indian villages as bedspreads. This will also suffice.

Posture During Meditation

This aspect is of great importance. All instructions in spiritual practice in India stress the importance of keeping the spine erect like a ramrod. The *Bhagavad Gita* says that the head, the neck and the spine should be in a single straight vertical line. Since subtle nerve currents flow through the bundle of nerves in the spinal cord and through the neck to the brain, it is important to keep them straight. (The spine should not be bent or crooked.) Further your breathing becomes easier and smoother, when your spine is erect.

In fact, the author can state with conviction that the practice of keeping the spine erect and the neck and the head in proper position during meditation will lead to better health and calmness in a few weeks. While doing this, the head and the neck should not be kept in a stiff, hard posture. Be as relaxed as you can. Those with slip disc or lower back pain or other deformities should not exert their spine. They can try to keep the spine erect and relaxed as much as possible and consult the orthopaedic physician for advice.

It is certainly possible to lie down on a flat, hard floor or mattress and meditate. The only problem is that one is likely to fall asleep!

Some use a Y-shaped chin support to hold the chin and keep their hand free for counting beads. Such practices are for well-trained yogis, who practise for several hours and not for a beginner or modern man who practises for short sessions.

Asanas During Meditation

Asana means *'seat'* and also the *posture* used for bending your limbs and other parts. In Hatha Yoga, asanas play a large part. For the meditator, however, simple sitting postures are recommended. Padmasana, or half Padma or Sukasan would be sufficient (Padma asan – Lotus posture). These asanas – in which your legs are tucked under the knees in a particular way – can be learnt easily. They help to sit firmly for long periods and to keep the spine erect, therefore their importance. If you cannot bend your knees easily or have difficulty in maintaining your asana, please do not get worried or feel diffident on that account. Meditation is more of mental practice. A physical posture or asana is of less importance.

Most meditators feel that after a few minutes of practise, they have a tendency to bend forward or lean to one side or bend backwards. Sometimes, as stresses are released, there is a tendency to oscillate or slightly shake towards the sides. These are normal reactions in the early days of practice. After about a month, such movements will stop. A meditator may feel very light; there may be a feeling of being lifted out of the seat. Please gently note such reactions. These are again normal reactions when nervous energy and 'prana' or life force are redirected.

During meditation, your blood pressure may decrease slightly. This may lead to a feeling of giddiness or swaying of the body. Such reactions decrease after a few days of practice. Some may experience slight headache in the first few days. This may again disappear after a few days of practice. If it persists, due to chronic migraine or other complaints, consult a doctor and reduce the duration of the meditation. After about a month of practice, such problems almost always disappear.

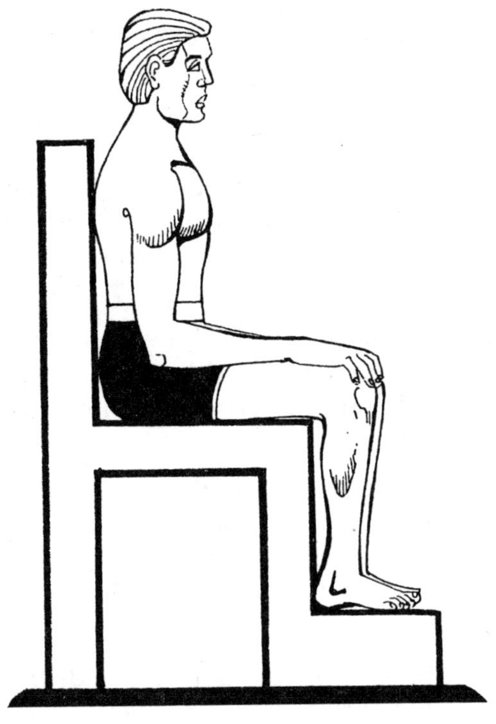

Fig. 1: Egyptian Statue Pose

Sitting Postures

Some westerners and those with knee problems would prefer doing meditation in a sitting posture in a chair. Again the back must be straight and may be supported by a backrest. Avoid the tendency to lean back. The posture suggested is called the Egyptian Statue Pose, as found at the entrance of the Great Pyramid (Fig 1). The feet should be firmly planted on the ground. The palms should be kept on the knees. The arms may be supported on the thighs. Practise sitting in the posture for a few minutes before starting meditation. Sit in the suggested posture and slowly breathe. Watch your breathing for 2 to 3 minutes. This practice in itself will give you much relaxation.

Position of Hands and Fingers – the Mudras

The position of hands and fingers assume great importance. Subtle nervous currents pass through our palms and fingers. (Those practising Reiki know the importance of the use of palms as channels for cosmic energy.) The hand signs are called *mudras* in Sanskrit and are used for symbolic communication in Indian (classical) dance forms.

In meditation, however, mudras indicate your mental states. According to the present writer, the best way to learn the hand signs is to study the Buddhist pictures and images, particularly the hand positions of Lord Buddha and Bodhisattvas.

The simplest mudra is to keep the palm of one hand over the palm of the other hand, both palms turned upwards. Keep the hands at the centre of the body, close to your navel. Some prefer to keep the palms on their thighs, turned upwards.

Others prefer to keep the fingers crossed, the tips of the fingers projecting forward like a steeple. Those studying body language have made deep analysis of such finger positions.

In one mudra, the hand is shown towards the ground and touching the seat. Lord Buddha was asked once: "Are you a celestial being? Have you come from the Heavens?"

Lord Buddha replied: "I am of this Earth" and showed this mudra, touching the ground. This mudra is therefore used to indicate basic feelings arising during meditation indicating that 'we are in touch with reality'.

Another common mudra for the contemplative state is as follows: Touch the thumb and index finger. The other fingers are outstretched. This is called 'contemplative mudra' or mudra used for teaching or instruction by a Master (chin mudra). This mudra indicates the annihilation of one's ego or ahamkara or 'I-ness'.

Note: *An important aspect of mudras during meditation is to be noted. For most meditators, the initial mudra at the start of the meditation is a voluntary act. He or she thinks of a particular mudra to assume during the practice. But while meditating the mudra may alter without a conscious act of the meditator. The present author has experienced this several times. It shows that the mind automatically (involuntarily) changes the mudra according to its state. In that sense, mudras are reflections of the mental state of the meditator. This is the reason for the great importance of mudras in Buddhist iconography. When a person returns to a normal state after meditation, he may be surprised to find his mudra had changed during the meditative session.*

In general, mudras help conserve nervous energy. Subtle currents pass through our fingers and jump from one finger to another like magnetic lines of force between poles of a magnet.

It is possible that ancient rishis and sages communicated certain messages through mudras during long sessions of meditation and *mouna* or silence. It was quite common for sages and seers to remain in silence for months and years. In our own times, Meher Baba remained silent for nearly 40 years, until his samadhi.

Hatha Yoga Practices

Hatha yoga practitioners use several different asanas or postures for physical and mental health. Among these asanas, Vajrasana or Simhasana (sitting postures) can also be used during meditation. But one need not strain oneself to practise these. Some yogis are known to do meditation or *tapas* (penance) standing on one leg. Some devotees do pooja or worship for Lord Shiva standing on one leg. Some use Vrikshasan (tree) pose for meditation. Such asana practise certainly improves the ability to concentrate on a single subject and boosts physical stamina. But they are of less importance to a meditator.

These are mentioned here as some teachers may advocate them. The present author would caution anyone in attempting these asanas. Physical frames of men and women these days are rarely adaptable for such strenuous practices. You may leave them for a few strong yogis in special ashrams or caves.

5. The Breath-watch

The breathing process controls the functioning of our vital organs – the heart and lungs – and indirectly our nervous system. In their own way, the Hindu seers discovered the subtle flow of energy though the nerves controlled by the breath. They found out the intricate relationship between the nerve nodes in the spinal cord and other locations called 'chakras' and the breathing process. It is through the various nodes of nerves that other physiological and mental processes are controlled. They also learnt how the endocrine glands could be regulated by attention to the nodes.

We are interested in the process of controlling the mind through the breath. How does one control the thought process through attention to the breath? This is an important step in our meditation.

It is common experience that when we are mentally agitated, angry or anxious, we breathe fast and hard. The reverse can be attempted. If we breathe slowly, deeply and gently, our mind would become calm and less agitated. We would feel rested. Deep, rhythmic breathing – even taking three or four breaths with full attention – can bring instant relief from our tensions and calm our mind.

(According to Hindu scriptures, the total lifespan of a person is determined by the number of breaths, not on chronological or calendar time.)

In meditation, however, our aim is a little deeper. Through breath-watch, we want to control our thoughts and seek quietness. To do this, a simple technique can be followed.

This technique is practised both by yogic masters and Zen meditation groups in slightly different forms.

Practice 2

- Sit in the usual meditative posture. Take a few deep breaths (3 or 4 times).
- Gently close the eyes; relax your legs and hands; relax your neck, shoulders and facial muscles.
- Focus your mind on the ingoing breath through the nostrils and the outgoing breath through the nostrils.

Note: *Do not count the number of breaths. Do not breathe forcefully faster or slower. Do not control the breath by holding or retaining after inhalation.*

Breathing should be natural, slow and smooth. Just watch the breath.

By doing this, you are not allowing your mind to dwell on other thoughts. You are directing your mind to your natural process. This frees your mind from the whirl of thoughts it normally engages in.

You can practise this with eyes open also; but it is easier when you close the eyes.

Just watch the breath as it goes in and goes out.

Initially you practise this for only five minutes; gradually, over a period of two to three weeks, increase it to 20 minutes. This practice alone will lead to calmness.

You can practise this at odd moments also, when you are travelling, waiting for a bus or train, or in a doctor's office.

Practise this at least twice a day. After a few days of practice, you will experience a sense of calmness and a new sense of freedom, not easily expressed in words. Nervous tension will be reduced. As thoughts are reduced, you will be able to think more calmly and act with deeper meaning attached to even simple actions. You will automatically be able to reduce activities of a trivial nature. You may also become less angry with others, as well as more tolerant and flexible in your approach.

(In traditional Zen schools, students practise this meditation for several hours. But that may not be possible for lay people with professional work. You can try longer periods on holidays.)

Walking Meditation

A variation of Breath-watch is the walking meditation – walk in gentle steps while watching the breath. You can do this in a garden, park or front porch or verandah of your house. Do this without talking to anybody, but just watching the ingoing and outgoing breath. You should do this at least for five minutes in one session, then take rest and again do this for the next five minutes. This practice at night before you retire to bed is very relaxing and will induce deep sleep. (Avoid doing this meditation when you are hungry or when your stomach is full after a heavy meal.)

Try this in your garden or in an open yard or in a beach on a full-moon day!

Breath-watch and walking meditations are excellent means to reduce daily stress.

Problems in Breath-watch

1. While doing breath-watch, thoughts will intrude, but gently put them away.
2. Avoid distractions like phone calls and avoid answering the doorbell.
3. Feel the coolness of your lungs. Don't force your breathing. Normally one breathes 15 or 16 times in a minute. In five minutes of practice, you will be watching nearly 80 breaths. This gives adequate quietness of mind.
4. If you feel shortness of breath, stop watching or walking, sit calmly or lie down.

6. Deep Breathing

This is accomplished by 'diaphragm breathing'. The *diaphragm* is *the muscle that separates the chest from the abdomen*. In this method, we make the diaphragm move freely up and down.

Deep breathing revitalises your body. You will feel refreshed and energetic. But do not overdo it. In the initial stages, practise for two to three minutes, twice or thrice a day. Note that an average person breathes 15 to 16 times a minute. Do not increase or decrease this number during deep breaths.

Practice 3

Raise the breastbone or sternum, keep it raised, and breathe out. Then, slowly breathe in and push the diaphragm down. It will take some time to get into this practice. After all, your breathing has been shallow and restricted for several years now. It is not going to change in a few days of practice. But keep practising, and you will feel positive benefits in a few weeks.

Practise for two to three minutes each time, twice or thrice a day. You can practise deep breaths when you feel tired or tense. Stand in front of an open window or in an open yard and practise.

Long Exhalation

This practice is to enable long and full exhalation by contracting the lungs and uplifting the diaphragm. The excess air should be expelled with some force while breathing out. You have to relax the muscles of your chest while doing this practice.

One famous yoga teacher would demonstrate this breathing out using a microphone with a long swishing sound or whistle-like blowing through the mouth.

In the early stages, it is all right to breathe out through the mouth. But in the later stages, breathing out should be through the nostrils.

Practice 4

Breathing out is connected with relaxing or the 'letting go' feeling. Develop proper feeling to enable complete exhalation, as you do while yawning... Only then can you breathe in fully. The stale air should be ejected. (For some people, especially those with asthmatic complaints, breathing out may be difficult. But regular practise of three to four breaths at a time would help. Asthmatics may realise that breathing out is dependent upon their feeling and thinking.) If a person feels relaxed and 'lets go', then he would find it easy to breathe out fully.

One method is to count one-two-three while breathing out. Check the number. Use the same number or count for breathing in. Once breathing in and breathing out are balanced, you will feel calm and mentally relaxed.

After some practise of balancing, try a longer exhalation, that is, breathing out should be a larger count than breathing in. A simple thumb-rule is that breathing out should be about 50% greater than breathing in. For instance, if you count 10 during breathing in, you should prolong breathing out to a count of 15.

After this practice, you can stretch your arms and yawn if you like.

Left and Right Channels

Ancient yogis clearly distinguished between breathing in through the left nostril and through the right nostril. This is perhaps connected with activating the left hemisphere or the right hemisphere of our brain separately. The left brain is related to dynamic activities and the outer world. The right brain is related to mental/cognitive activities, reflections and inner perception. Modern psychologists have probed right brain and left brain thinking a great deal.

For most of us, one part of the brain, either left or right, is more activated or energised than the other. This leads to the mental tendency of humans being introverts or extroverts. It is important to achieve balance in the activation of the left and right brain. Through a simple process of Pranayama, yogis teach us to achieve this balance. (*Prana* is the *life force*; it also refers to nerve currents flowing through the nerves in different parts of the body; *ayama* means *regulation*, often also translated as *'control'*.)

Practice 5

With the middle finger or index finger, press and close one of the nostrils, say the left one. Now slowly breathe in and breathe out with the right nostril. Next, close the right nostril, and breathe in and out through the left nostril. You can practise this three or four times.

In the second step, close the left nostril and breathe in through the right nostril. After complete inhalation, close the right nostril with the index finger and breathe out through the left nostril. The next time, you reverse the process by breathing in through the left and breathing out through the right. This practice is called reverse breathing. Repeat this practice three or four times only. **Do not practise this more than four times in one session.**

> **Note:** *Many persons are first sceptical about the whole theory of single nostril breathing. It is hard to prove its efficacy scientifically, and the present author is not aware of scientific studies on this aspect. But a practising meditator would find the results through increased mental strength and clarity of mind.*

7. Meditative Practices – Preliminary Steps

We have discussed the important breathing practices associated with meditation. Before we consider the mental processes of meditation, we shall describe a few preliminary steps normally practised by Hindu meditators. Similar steps are used in other traditions. You may vary the steps according to your particular religious or spiritual traditions.

1. Start with Invocation

Pray to God or the Almighty or your favourite deity (Ishta Devata) or guru (living or dead) to help you with the meditation: Lord ________, I pray to Thee to calm my mind and shower Your blessings and assist me in performing this meditation. (Many Hindus will offer a prayer to Lord Ganesha.)

2. Mention Specific Requests or Prayers or Healing Needs

This is called *'sankalpa'* or your resolve to get help for specific needs. Be as specific as you can:

"I seek Lord ________'s help in healing my body from the ailment of ________.

"I seek Lord ________'s help in performing well in the forthcoming oral examination."

"I seek Lord ________'s help towards better understanding of the scripture ________ I am studying now."

> **Note:** *If you feel uncomfortable with seeking such specific help from the Cosmic Power, you may skip this step.*

3. Make Positive Affirmations

Affirmations are statements made with the full belief that what we want is already given to us or accomplished. Make affirmations in the present tense:

"I affirm that I am healed of my knee swellings."

"I affirm that I have made a great presentation to my Board members."

"I affirm that I devote my time and energy to fulfil the tasks for my schoolchildren."

"I affirm that I have overcome this problem of misunderstanding with my spouse."

Repeat the affirmation thrice to imprint it in your mind. In reality, affirmations are messages given to your subconscious mind. The subconscious mind works almost 24 hours of the day, without your conscious intervention.

Mind Focus

A major task in meditation is to achieve a level of concentration not obtained by many people in the ordinary run of daily work. Our thoughts jump from one topic to another or from one work to another. This processing of endless thoughts fritters away a lot of energy. Our scriptures give the analogy that our mind is like a drunken monkey, bitten by a scorpion, jumping from one branch of a tree to another!

The focused mind can be likened to a laser beam, a coherent, parallel shaft of light, which causes very little dispersion or spreading even when projected on a wall several feet away, with very little divergence. Ordinary light from your torch will form a large circle of light with dimness.

One yogi wrote that the great battle of meditation is with restless thoughts. Only when the thoughts quieten down in meditation, and you concentrate on the Divine Being, can you reach Him.

Practice 6: The Practice of NOW!

It is important to learn to keep your thinking restricted to the present.... Now, Now, NOW! For the next five minutes, scrupulously avoid any thought of the past, the past hour, yesterday, last year or several years ago... You will realise how difficult it becomes. But once you are aware of your thoughts jumping to the past, you can exercise control over such thoughts. Practise for five minutes at a time, three or four times a day.... This is indeed a great practice. Motivate yourself by saying that such past thoughts are irrelevant or useless or a drain on your energy.

There are moments when you can indulge in your past thoughts – moments of nostalgic memories when you meet your old friend or visit your native place or old school. These are, of course, rare moments. Except on such occasions, you should avoid past thoughts. You will then have plenty of time to do other things.

It is common observance that as you grow older, especially after you cross 50 years, your thoughts will be more on your past than on your present or the future. It requires considerable effort to plan and dream about the future, and yet you must do that at times.

Past thoughts, both pleasant and unpleasant, are wasted energy. According to Yoga and Vedanta (a school of Hindu philosophy), only the present is REAL; the past and the future are unreal and part of our ignorance or *'avidya'*.

One may feel that it is difficult to think of the present only. Consider this situation. You are a bank officer in real life. But, as a member of an amateur drama club, you go to the stage and play the role of Anthony in the Shakespearean play *Anthony and Cleopatra*. While you are acting, you think about your role only and the words you have to speak and the gestures to make. You would not think about what you had done in the bank yesterday or what you have to do tomorrow. Likewise, it is possible to live in the present most of the time.

(Most self-development books and management-oriented books emphasise planning for the future. This has relevance in a certain context; for instance, you must plan for your retirement from active work. Except in such cases, YOU MUST BE IN THE PRESENT. Self-help books rarely discuss the thinking of the present, as they assume that we all do that! Dale Carnegie, however, in his inimitable all-time classic *How to Stop Worrying and Start Living* emphasised living in day-tight compartments in the very first chapter! Thinking of only today's work and problems is a definite step towards mental health. Not enough! Thinking about this moment allows you to control your mind through its REAL nature – a discovery made by ancient Hindu seers.)

In fact, the very purpose of 'breath-watch' is to focus on the present and give a respite to your mind which most of the time thinks about the past.

(A major part of Zen meditation is devoted to practising thinking of this moment, whether you are walking, eating, speaking or taking bath.)

Practice 7: Awareness Listening

A related practice is as follows. Sit calmly in your garden or a public park or beach. Do not read or speak to anyone. Do not make any gestures to anyone. Just move your head and calmly observe the things in the garden for five minutes. Focus only on the things in front of your eyes. Avoid all extraneous thoughts... Then gently close your eyes. Listen to all the sounds – try focusing on the sounds, both pleasant and unpleasant... Then take deep breaths four times... Focus on the smells from plants, flowers, animals and insects. Feel the air rubbing over your skin.

Note: *This practice will impart calmness and improve the acuteness of your senses. The present author had experienced this effectively when he could hear the passage of a distant train – about 2 km away – in the heart of a city at 9 PM with several intervening large apartment buildings.*

8. Concentrating on Your Life Force or Prana

With the practise of breathing exercises explained earlier, you may reach the stage of controlling your life force or *prana* and directing prana to specific parts of the body. This direction of prana helps in two ways:

1. To relax and rejuvenate that part of the body and
2. To heal that part if it is functionally deranged or damaged.

Note that reaching this stage is an important and critical step in your progress chart. *It is a milestone of progress and should be recognised as such.* Some may attain this stage after a month or two, while some may require a year or more of serious practise. Many may give up meditation before reaching this stage for they see no 'definite' or 'specific' improvement till then and only experience certain degrees of mental relaxation or decrease in mental tension. But, after you reach the stage of control of prana, you are literally 'hooked on' to meditation for life. Since some do take a long time to reach this stage, one should continue these techniques at least for a year before giving up or changing your views on these techniques.

We shall explain briefly the method of directing your prana or life force towards specific parts of the body. Normally, depending on the usage and healthy condition of various parts, prana may be directed to various parts without your knowledge. For instance, an intellectual person will have more prana flowing into his brain. On the other hand, a car mechanic will have more prana flowing to his hands and legs, which he uses more. After a meal, more prana flows into your stomach region. But it is possible that one overuses some part without giving rest or enough prana to that part. In course of time that part gets deranged or one feels terribly tired or becomes totally dysfunctional. Redirecting prana is a conscious effort.

When one redirects prana to a specific part, he can see tangible sensations; for instance, that part becomes warm or even quite hot or, sometimes, rather cool. It is possible for your leg muscles and knees to become warm, or your head to become cool. (Yes, indeed, we want a 'cool' head and 'warm' feet.) Before a major decision, you may meditate and direct your prana to the head so that it becomes really 'cool' and then you may proceed to discuss the matter.

Practice 8: Directing Prana

1. Sit in a meditative posture.
2. Practise breath-watch for five minutes.
3. Close your eyes and think of the part to be energised.
4. Make a '*sankalpa*' or affirmation: "I energise this part with my prana."
5. Concentrate your mind on that part and relax to feel the sensation in that part.
6. Continue concentrating for 5 to 10 minutes. (Initially do this only for two to three minutes.)
7. Practise breath-watch again.
8. Open your eyes and take a few sips of water or fruit juice.

> **Note:** *This practice is quite difficult for a beginner. Persistence helps. If a teacher or guru guides you, it becomes easier and the progress more rapid, since a teacher can listen to your problems and give suggestions towards a solution. It is important to master the earlier practices before you begin this practice.*

Withdrawing the Senses

In Patanjali's eight-part or eight-limbed yoga, *Ashtanga Yoga* (*Ashta = eight* and *anga = part*), one of the parts is called 'PRATYAHARA'. This is withdrawing your mind from the senses running towards their objects. For instance, our eyes are attracted towards various things and then curiosity or desire arises; with desire, some action may follow. This yoga step is basically intended to silence the sense organs.

> **Note:** *Raja Yoga, for which Patanjali's Yoga aphorisms (sutras) form the basic text, is an extremely complicated subject. We shall not dwell on this in a general book of this kind. There are several books in English on this subject, which are either oversimplified or incorrect interpretations in many respects. The reader may read the books referred to in the 'Select Bibliography', which are excellent texts. This subject should preferably be learnt from a master who has personal experience of the various stages of this yoga and not from mere Sanskrit scholars or philosophers with limited or mistaken views.*

Our mind runs after objects of the senses. For instance, if your eyes see an interesting advertisement on TV, your mind is attracted and dwells on the item advertised; a desire may arise that you should possess that item and you may rush to send a cheque. We are constantly titillated by visual images.

Objects of other senses also attract us – we may like some music or fine smell in the garden. Withdrawal from all these sense objects is part of meditation practice.

Considerable control over the senses is essential for all meditators and spiritual seekers. Do the practise gradually, since the senses are not easy to control. If you forcibly shut yourself up in an isolated room, you may develop depression or be invaded by past ugly, painful thoughts. Therefore, practise only for a few minutes at each session. Gradually reduce the time you spend watching TV, or listening to the radio or reading magazines and newspapers. Avoid street noise or construction site noise or loud music. Soft music can soothe your nerves and induce better sleep, but again do not overdo it or get addicted to certain types of music. Pratyahara should be practised in a balanced and sensible way.

Yoga literature usually compares this process of pratyahara to the withdrawal of limbs by a tortoise. The limbs are drawn inwards, and its shell covers the tortoise. Keep this image in mind when you practise withdrawal of the senses.

Apart from meditative sessions, you can practise this in other moments – for instance, while travelling on a long-distance train or bus or waiting at a railway station or airport. Advanced yogis can practise this even in a crowded noisy place.

Intense Viewing

You can increase your power of concentration by intense viewing – look at a particular spot or item. You may blink or close the eyes when tired or when the eyes water.

The spot for concentration may be a mountaintop or a church tower or a beach at a distance in the open countryside. In your altar room or pooja room or meditation hall, set up a picture or image or idol at the eye level. Keep a simple background and soft or diffused light in the room. You may keep a lighted candle at the eye level and practise intense viewing. Take in as much detail as possible of the object.

During devotional practice in Hindu homes, we intensely observe the feet or the hands of the Lord's picture or image. One should develop a sense of humility when concentrating. This practice may precede chanting prayers or hymns. At the advanced level, intense viewing leads to a high degree of concentration and mental surrender at the feet of the Lord, as a humble servant or slave of the Lord. Such traditions exist in almost all religions and is an important step in pratyahara. You may practise this for five to 30 minutes in the early stages.

Note: *Those who experience chronic eye problems or migraine headaches or epilepsy should consult a doctor before practising this intense viewing.*

This practice is different from autohypnosis, since a person is constantly aware that he is viewing an external object.

9. Words and Mantras

After sufficient practise on breathing as given earlier, say, after a month, the meditator can go to the next step of associating a word or mantra with breathing in and out.

The word *'mantra'* has acquired an esoteric or mystical meaning to many, particularly among westerners. Mantras are specially chosen or selected syllables to be used during meditation. While one may chose one's own mantra, as we shall suggest later, usually the mantras are given by a guru or preceptor during a formal ceremony or ritual called *'Mantra Diksha'* or initiation.

This initiation is to invoke the gods first, then one's guru or the guru's lineage – a succession of gurus called *'Guru Parampara'* – and then to give the mantra after perhaps certain practise to arouse pranic energy. To many not familiar with such traditions, this ritual may appear as mumbo-jumbo or trickery, to create a certain mystery or aura around the process or be taken merely as a means of making money. While there are many bogus gurus to fleece money from the gullible, this process has sound basis in Yoga, called Mantra Yoga, and is also part of Laya Yoga or Tantric cults.

For most beginners, however, simple, common mantras are all that is necessary. Only these are advocated in this book, though one may choose to follow a guru of one's choice.

The most useful and potent mantra in Hindu tradition is OM or AUM. It consists of three syllables: A for creation, U for preservation and M for destruction or dissolution, which are the roles of the major gods – Brahma, Vishnu and Shiva.

There are volumes written on this mantra, with a variety of interpretations. Several Upanishads, especially the *Mandukya Upanishad,* elaborate on the significance of this mantra. It is also extolled in the *Bhagavad Gita*. This mantra has cosmological significance too, since it is associated with the creation of the Cosmos. This mantra is called 'PRANAVA' and is accepted by all sects in the Hindu religion as a sacred mantra.

Practice 9: Chanting OM

Sit in the usual meditative posture. Take three or four deep breaths. Watch the breath for one minute (15 or 16 breaths).

Then chant AUM slowly; it should be audible, but not loud. It should not be a faint murmur. You can exhale through the mouth if you feel out of breath.

Chant nine times or in multiples of nine. Normally one is advised to chant 108 times or in multiples of 108 or 1008 times.

If you chant 216 times, that will constitute just 1% of the number of breaths per day. (Normally a person breathes 15 times a minute and, therefore, the total number of breaths per day is 15 x 60 x 24 = 21,600. The present author believes that any mantra chanting should be repeated at least for 1% of the breathing process, i.e., 216 times.)

Note that "A" is pronounced with drawing of the breath, "U" is with a swishing sound or like whistling, and "M" with a gentle closing of the mouth. It is also stated that the tongue should not touch the palate. With a little practise, one can chant "A-U-M" effortlessly.

Other Mantras

Several mantras are available in common practice. Usually they are extensions of OM.

You attach God's names with Om, for instance, OM Ram, OM SAI, or OM Bhavani

More elaborate mantras are: 'OM Namo Narayana', which means, *Om, I bow to Narayana* (*Ashtakshari* or 8-syllabled one). Likewise, Shiva worshippers chant 'Om Namah Shivaya' (*Panchakshari* or 5-syllabled one). A more elaborate mantra is: 'OM Maha Ganapathi Namah', in honour of Lord Ganesha.

In Buddhist schools, a famous mantra is 'Om Mani Padme Ham' which means, *I invoke the jewel or gem in the lotus.* One is supposed to meditate on the navel or Manipura chakra and chant this. Manipura chakra at the navel region is the seat of creation. Manipura literally means 'City of Gems'. Lord Brahma, the creator, emanates from the navel of Lord Vishnu. This form of meditation can lead to mental peace and, in later stages, to a feeling of detachment.

The present author has had some experience with this meditation, the details of which cannot be given in a general book of this kind. (Some authors write that this chanting is done with meditation on the heart – anahata – chakra, which is not correct. There are specific mantras for each chakra, as we shall discuss in a later chapter.)

Practice 10: Mantra and Breathing

While chanting these mantras, one learns to associate the syllables with breathing in and out steps. For instance, one breathes in with the syllable OM and utters *Shivaya* while breathing out. Such steps are easy to learn and may become automatic after some practice.

It is also okay to chant within the mind without uttering audible syllables. This requires much practise and can be used by advanced meditators.

Note: *This subject of meditating with mantras is a subtle process and one should practise at least for a month to realise its value.*

SOHAM Meditation

This is an advanced Advaitic (non-dual, monistic) tradition meditation. Only those who are fairly advanced, and who have studied Advaitic philosophy and subscribe to it, should practise this. Otherwise, using this meditation is cheating oneself. This philosophy of Advaita or monism is well established and several books and websites on this exist. It derives its strength from the Vedas. Adi Shankara (AD 788–820) was the main exponent of this philosophy, after Buddhism dealt a great blow to Hindu faith. In a sense, Adi Shankara resurrected this philosophy and placed it on firm foundations based on the Upanishads. (There are controversies about the dates of Adi Shankara while this one – AD 788 to 820 – is widely accepted.) More recent masters of Advaita were Bhagwan Ramana Maharshi (Thiruvannamalai, Tamil Nadu) and Nisargadatta Maharaj (Mumbai) who are no more with us.

SO-HAM stands for 'I am He', in which the individual soul or Jiva in each of us asserts oneness with the Supreme Being, Brahman or He, pervading the Universe. (This is the basic tenet of Advaita in a single sentence!) (Sah – He means Brahman, Aham – Jiva or one's Soul.) While breathing in, one chants 'SO' and while breathing out, chant 'Ham'. There are variations in some schools of Yoga.

Many meditators are taught this meditation, which is highly efficacious. Only practise will convince you. The present author pursued this path, with some variation, for nearly 12 years. (He also practised this at a young age for a few months and then left due to the tremendous surge of energy.) At one time he felt that no other meditation practice is required except this, such is its power. Now he feels that even SOHAM meditation is a bit difficult and other methods stated earlier are easier to practise and could be highly effective for many householders.

Some yogis, however, state that this is only a preliminary step and there are other more potent techniques. The present author can only remark based on his personal experience and cannot argue about other notions or views taken from other teachers or books.

Note: *There are other schools of Vedanta, like Vishista Advaita or qualified monism, established by Sri Ramanuja (AD 1077–1197) and pure duality or Dvaita of Sri Madhva, and other acharyas like Nimbarka, Vallabha and Sri Chaitanya Mahaprabhu. We shall not digress into these topics, but only state that Soham meditation refers to pure monism of the Adi Shankara school.*

If one practices Soham meditation well and attains sufficient mastery, it should be considered a major milestone in progress. Many may not go beyond this or may deviate into other paths such as that of devotion or Bhakti Yoga or pure Gyana and give up meditation altogether. Nothing definite can be said about such deviations – it is like the career change of a person in the mundane world. In the final analysis, it all depends on one's own destiny (*'prarabda'*) or the guru's grace!

Meditation of Loving Kindness

This meditation is similar to the famous Buddhist meditation, 'mitta'. It is also often practised in groups.

In this, the meditator sends out affirmations for the health and happiness of other people, with 'loving kindness.'

Practice 11: Loving Kindness

First start with Breath-watch for five minutes. Chant gently as follows:

While breathing in, say to yourself: "May I be well."

While breathing out, say to yourself: "May others be well."

Repeat this at least four times.

Lengthen the breathing out; visualise people of different countries, races, colours, and age groups at that time.

Lengthen the breathing out; visualise spiritual masters: Lord Buddha, Jesus Christ, Prophet Mohammed, Chaitanya Mahaprabhu, Sri Ramakrishna Paramahansa, Bhagwan Ramana Maharshi, Shirdi Sai Baba and so on.

Lengthen breathing out; visualise your close relations, teachers, friends, and workers.

Focus on your heart and say: "May I be well, may others be well."

(Some imagine a flower or lotus in the heart region.)

Practise this meditation in the morning at dawn and before retiring to bed.

10. Chakra Meditation and Healing

Auras and Chakras

Our body is encased in a thin sheath of light called *aura*. This aura is invisible to our eyes, but can be photographed by a special technique called Kirlian Photography, named after a Russian electrician and mystic, Semyon Kirlian (1900–1980). The aura may extend to a few feet from our body. It may be coloured light. Near some parts of the body, the aura may be thin while it may be dense near other portions of the body. An auric healer may be able to see your aura and from its deficiency, infer your physical condition or disease. The reader should consult special books on this subject. Some mystics and meditators may have their auras extended over several metres.

Chakra is a Sanskrit word for *wheel* and came to represent a nervous bundle that may send out waves or prana (life force). They are like electrical distribution transformers you find in any big city. Some transformers are large and some small. Likewise, we have several chakras in our body, major and minor ones. Some claim 40 or 72 chakras, but for our discussion we focus on 10 major chakras.

Of the ten, seven chakras are situated in our spinal column and play the greatest role. In addition, we have two important chakras in our palms and one major chakra near the spleen. Some would include the chakras at the inner palm of our feet in this list.

Hindu Yogis and Tantrics attach importance to the seven chakras. Energy flows out of these chakras through various nerves, and they regulate and control endocrine glands close to them. We shall discuss the details later.

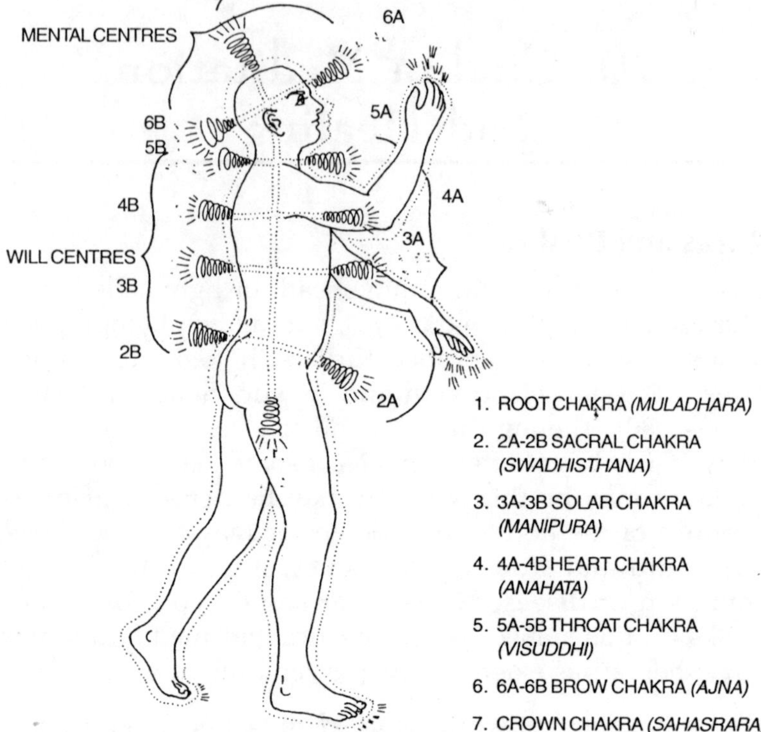

1. ROOT CHAKRA *(MULADHARA)*
2. 2A-2B SACRAL CHAKRA *(SWADHISTHANA)*
3. 3A-3B SOLAR CHAKRA *(MANIPURA)*
4. 4A-4B HEART CHAKRA *(ANAHATA)*
5. 5A-5B THROAT CHAKRA *(VISUDDHI)*
6. 6A-6B BROW CHAKRA *(AJNA)*
7. CROWN CHAKRA *(SAHASRARA)*

Fig. 2: The Major Chakras

According to Tantra, two important nerves called *Ida* (left side) and *Pingala* (the right side) are twisted around the spinal cord. They are also referred to as moon (cool) nadi or nerve and sun (hot) nadi or nerve. Nervous energy, which is only a form of prana, flows up or down these nerves at a given time and keeps our body healthy and energetic.

At the centre, in the middle of the spinal cord is a vertical nerve called *Sushumna*. This being very thick, to carry a large flow of energy like a thick cable, it is a bundle of thin nerves, and referred to as a 'channel'. We can better appreciate it as a thick optical cable, as used by telephone engineers. Light energy may flow through this and some yogis refer to this as a silvery blue luminescent nerve, quite like an optical fibre!

In Yoga literature, it is stated that this sushumna is normally closed and by certain yogic practices, it is pierced so that spiritual nectar can flow up the channel to the brain or the Sahasrara chakra. All this is a pictorial way of describing the flow of energy to the brain centre, as if a fluid is injected up a hollow tube. In modern terminology, we can understand it in terms of an optical cable carrying energy and information to the head. It is better we avoid the concept of a liquid moving up the channel, as mentioned in traditional literature. The sushumna is normally not activated. Yogic practices help to open up this channel, that is, to send energy and information by a kind of switch we do not understand as of now.

The Seven Major Chakras

The seven major chakras, located along the spinal column, are:

MULADHARA – base chakra, also means foundation chakra, at the base of the spine near the anal region. This is also called 'earth' chakra.

SŴADHISTHANA – at the sacral region near the genitals.

MANIPURA – (the city of gems or jewels) at the navel region, near the solar plexus.

ANAHATA – at the heart region – anahata also refers to the sound heard in the heart region – '*anahata*' means *eternal* or *supernal.*

VISUDDHI – purified – at the throat region, between the thyroid glands.

AJNA – literally means '*command*' – at the point between the eyebrows.

SAHASRARA – thousand-petalled, also called crown chakra, near the pineal gland, in the brain.

In yogic and tantric literature, each chakra is associated with a flower with certain number of petals and a colour. The petals are used to remember the syllables of the mantra associated with that chakra. The yogi meditates on the lotus, imagining its colour. When the chakra is not activated, the lotus has petals hanging down. While the chakra is activated, the flower becomes upturned with petals pointing upwards.

Note that these are symbolic ways of describing purely mental processes and a way to help remember things. In ancient India, when these concepts were developed, books were not written. Young students had to remember what their tutors told them. They had to repeat what was told and pictorially absorb and remember the details, hence all these imaginative symbolic representation of chakras. The details of chakras were also engraved in stones, usually kept in temples. A beginner need not burden himself with much of the details given in Tantra books, which are of limited use to a meditator.

The Kundalini

The following spiritual interpretation is, however, important. Kundalini is the cosmic energy, worshipped as a Hindu universal goddess. She is supposed to be like a coiled serpent at the base of the spine at the Muladhara chakra. Due to yogic practices or intense devotion, the coiled serpent is supposed to rise, piercing each chakra going from the Muladhara to the Swadhisthana, then to the next one, Manipura and so on.

(In Hindu tradition, we associate a symbolic goddess with many things. For instance, rivers like Ganga are worshipped as goddesses. Likewise, this nadi or nerve channel is mystically termed a goddess.)

The ascent of this Kundalini, activating each chakra, is accompanied by new powers and abilities in the individual. For instance, when Kundalini reaches the throat (Visuddhi) chakra, one may start singing and writing poetry, even though the person might have been an illiterate. (Due to the activation of this chakra, many Indian poets like the great Kalidasa were suddenly gifted with poetic talent. The legends allude to persons receiving a special gift from the Goddess of Learning, Saraswathi. Prophet Mohammed received the inspiration and command from God to write poetry after penances.)

Finally, Kundalini reaches the Crown chakra or Sahasrara, which will cause an 'effulgence of thousand suns' or extreme brilliance, leading to cosmic vision (mentioned in the *Bhagavad Gita* – Chapter 11), as perceived by Arjuna at the instance of Lord Krishna and that would result in Self-Realisation or Liberation or Moksha. (There are several controversial descriptions or issues on this aspect.)

> **Note:** *The word* 'sahasra' *means* one thousand; *it should be noted that Vedic seers used this word to denote* 'innumerable' *or* infinite, *rather than just one thousand. This notion is found in many places, 'like thousand-faced purusha' or god in* 'Purusha Sukta' *in the Vedas. Therefore, the crown chakra has innumerable petals, often depicted by several petals in the head of the images of Lord Buddha.*

The allegory of Kundalini is furthered extended as follows: The ascent of the Kundalini and reaching the crown chakra is described as merging of Shakti, the Female Goddess with the all-powerful Purusha or the Male God or Shiva. This union of Shakti with Shiva constitutes the final culmination of spiritual progress.

How does the Kundalini rise from the Muladhara? Some authors contend that it moves up from one chakra to another, slowly. There could be several months or even years before it moves up one step. Others state that Kundalini raises quickly like quick-silver or mercury and it could be a matter of a few days or a few hours. The present author is not in a position to accept one view or the other. The experiences could vary for different practitioners. The author contends that through yoga it is possible to activate each and every chakra *separately* based on the particular mental and spiritual status. Sometimes more than one chakra may be opened up and become operative.

Role of Chakras

It is important to understand carefully the role of each chakra for worldly benefit and for one's own spiritual development. This discussion is necessarily brief because some of the esoteric concepts cannot be included in a general book of this kind.

It is easier to understand the roles of chakras by dividing them into two groups... the lower three (basal, sacral and navel – usually called physical chakras) and the upper three (throat, eyebrow and crown – usually called spiritual chakras) with the heart (anahata) chakra in the middle.

The middle one, the heart chakra, occupies a special place. Cosmic energy can be absorbed by this chakra and then distributed to the lower chakras or partly sent up, to the upper chakras. It acts as a valve to control the flow of energy. This, of course, is again a simplified way of describing the energy process. (In Reiki practice, some of these concepts are further developed and given specific procedures. The interested reader should refer to books on Reiki.)

Reference to Indian Mythology

A reader familiar with Hindu mythology and Puranic literature can understand certain aspects of Kundalini with the mythical symbols. The navel or Manipura chakra is associated with creative energies. According to Hindu mythology, Lord Vishnu holds the God of Creation, Brahma, from His navel centre on a lotus. The serpent Sesha with thousand hoods (*Ananta Nag*) protects Lord Vishnu. This may represent the Sahasrara chakra that protects the Lord.

In Buddhist literature, the focus is put on the Manipura chakra, which represents not only creativity, but denotes physical energy and longevity. They also refer to this chakra as *'hara'*. It is considered the seat of life, though we normally associate life with the heart. Buddhist monks meditate on the navel chakra with the chant *'Om Mani Padme Ham'*, as explained earlier. Such meditation can lead to increased appetite, physical strength and spiritual progress with gradual sense of detachment from worldly desires.

Warning Note on Kundalini Practice

There is a common misconception that a master can awaken Kundalini by a simple procedure for any person without paying attention to previous preparations and achieving a degree of mental purity or 'Chita Suddhi'. *This is to be discouraged. Such quick arousal of Kundalini, if at all possible, is dangerous and may do more harm than good to the individual.*

(There are yogis who believe in mass awakening of Kundalinis in a group of people in a single session. This author is of the opinion that such claims are often exaggerated to win large-scale following and to give the impression that such methods are easy and simple. He is unable to confirm or accept such claims.)

(There is a method of awakening the Kundalini by a master or guru, often referred to as *Shaktipath* in yogic literature. Several methods of initiation are included under this general title 'shaktipath' or the path of Goddess Shakti. Those interested may read books by Swami Muktananda of Ganeshpuri and his lineage of gurus... There is a similar line of tantric cult, especially in the south, following Sri Vidya Upasana or worship. This method is supposed to have been propagated by no less a person than the great monist Adi Shankara.)

Yogic literature is full of warnings on the practice of Pranayama and Kundalini Yoga since the possible damage to the physical organs and the brain are known in India. This is due to the fact that one learning the process on his own by self-help or bookish knowledge or guided by an inexperienced or misguided teacher or guru can practise in a wrong way. Furthermore, many have ruined their health due to overexertion in the early stages. But the simple techniques suggested here are quite safe.

One factor that should be kept in mind is the age of the person; many Pranayama or Kundalini exercises are to be practised from a young age. Those who have crossed 40 years must be careful about these practices and should consult a medical doctor and a competent teacher before starting any such practice. The author does not recommend the retention of breath during Pranayama for those above 40 years of age. Likewise, Pranayama with bellow-like breathing, called Bhastrika Pranayama (like a blacksmith's bellow to stoke the fire), should not be practised at all in modern times.

Gentle breathing practices outlined earlier and the calm meditation techniques are easy to use at any age. Awakening Kundalini or activating chakras by quick methods after an hour or two of initiation without any systematic meditation practice is harmful and should be avoided. The author is aware of some gurus who advocate quick and simplified paths to awaken Kundalini. These methods are, for the most part, ineffective and may prove dangerous. It is like passing a 11 kilovolt electric current from the main transmission line into your household electric wires. You know that the power supply should be reduced to 220 volts or 110 volts by step-down transformers before being sent into your house cables. Many practices of quick Kundalini awakening are like passing 11 KV current into your household system. In the over-enthusiasm to popularise their method and create a large following or collect large sums of money, some yogis have been teaching such methods. The author strongly advises the aspirant not to follow such methods.

Several preparatory steps, as given here, are required before taking to Kundalini Yoga. Breathing meditation and practise of SOHAM meditation for at least six months are required before attempting the work on chakras. Great masters like Paramahansa Yogananda always advised their disciples to practise chanting and follow devotional practices before getting into Kundalini awakening. A lot of self-discipline is required for any serious yoga practise. Individual instruction under the guidance of a master is the safest route and not mass instruction in a large hall.

Healing Through Chakras

Chakra healing is a specialised subject. We shall briefly present the main concepts. Any meditation process on the chakras leads to cleansing and healing of the body parts associated with that chakra.

Muladhara chakra gives physical and mental stability. It is important to work for long hours on this chakra before exercising other chakras. It helps in getting down-to-earth feelings. It will reduce fanciful thinking, wild imagination and bad dreams. As a result, your intuition will develop. At the physical level, it will improve your physical strength with increased appetite and assimilation. It helps to improve the ability to digest food and stabilises the metabolism. Many teachers pay attention only to this chakra for several months. This is also true of some Buddhist practices.

Swadhisthana or sacral chakra is associated with sex organs and thoughts related to sex, and emotional pleasure. This centre is also concerned with our social interactions and mental poise.

Manipura or navel chakra is connected with creative powers, digestive organs and impulses that lead to new activities and adventures. This centre can also lead to negative emotions such as anger and jealousy. Those who feel depressed often, or feel passive or disinterested in life, should activate this chakra through meditation. Tibetan Buddhist traditions attach much importance to this chakra, also called '*hara*', for healing. In daily life, one is supposed to keep this navel region relaxed and flexible.

Anahata or heart chakra is the seat of emotions and feelings towards others. As stated in religious literature, it is the place of compassion and love. Violent passions also arise from the heart chakra. From the yogic viewpoint, it is also the place of deep meditation in which the ego or *ahamkara* would subside and get dissolved in the heart before self-realisation. A state of egolessness is attained. Some refer to this chakra as a cave or inner chamber. Advanced yogis may hear specific sounds emanating from the heart centre. The heart centre is not the physical heart that is a pump. The heart is supposed to be in the exact centre of the chest, though some yogis point to other locations. Activating the heart centre is a major step in spiritual growth.

As already stated, the heart chakra divides the lower three chakras from the upper three and forms a storehouse for spiritual energy. This energy may be diverted to upper regions for yogis and towards lower chakras in worldly people occupied with mundane matters. Cosmic energy is drawn through the crown and passed onto the heart chakra for redistribution. (Hindus also believe that one's prana or life force leaves the body at the time of death through the crown for yogis. The soft portion of the crown where one maintains a tuft of hair is supposed to be the door into the crown.)

The heart chakra has to work closely with the throat chakra and eyebrow chakra for poetical, religious and spiritual impulses. A great yogi or saint is often a mystical poet and seer, *trikala gyani* (one with knowledge of the past, present and future). It is clear that all the three chakras must be fully activated for such states. A saint, in moments of spiritual ecstasy, may burst into song or hymns and may write sublime poems. (Prophet Mohammed, when inspired by Saint Gabriel, became an instant poet and wrote the Quranic verses within a short time. We may call this divine inspiration due to his penances.)

The heart chakra is also the seat of desires. We say 'my heartfelt desire'. Such strong desires may lead to actions that are not always ethical. Imbalance in this chakra leads to excessive desires, anger (due to frustration caused by unfulfilled desires) and tendency for possessiveness and greed. These are the major vices, often mentioned in Vedanta, namely *kama* (desire), *krodha* (anger) and *madha* (greed and arrogance). One who eschews these three vices is well on the road to spiritual progress. The practice is to meditate on this chakra with thoughts of well-being and happiness for all people on Earth. (*'Sarva jana sukhino bhavantu'* meaning, "Let all people be in peace and joy".)

Visuddhi or throat chakra is the seat of expression, word power and poetry. One who has this chakra activated is articulate, highly communicative and sociable. At higher levels, he or she becomes a preacher, expounding sublime truths – a preceptor or religious leader. While some religious leaders choose to remain quiet and practise silence (like Bhagwan Ramana and Meher Baba who only answered questions put to them) some are given to lecturing and *prachar*, wandering through various places spreading their doctrines. Gautama Buddha, Adi Shankara, Swami Vivekananda, Swami Rama Tirtha and, in our own times, Swami Chinmayananda and Bhakti Vedanta Prabhupada (of the Hare Krishna movement) are perfect examples of sadhus in the preaching mode. We can surmise that their visuddhi chakras were fully developed and active.

(A digression here. It is interesting to note that all these great sadhus travelled widely through the length and breadth of India and some of them extensively toured foreign countries as well. The tremendous energies exhibited by them were due to the awakening of their Visuddhi, Muladhara and Manipura chakras. Some of them travelled when they were very young, like Swami Vivekananda and Adi Shankara, while Swami Chinmaya and Srila Prabhupada travelled even in advanced years. When Prabhupada went to New York to preach for the first time, he was 69 years old! But one should not pass judgment on sadhus only on this ability. Some like Bhagwan Ramana Maharishi, Shirdi Sai Baba and Nisargadatta Maharaj never moved out of their ashrams or homes. We can also note that the former category established an order of monks, while the latter group (Bhagwan Ramana, Shirdi Sai Baba, Nisargadatta among others) did not have appointed or anointed gurus or pontiffs in their line! Such are the various kinds of gurus of traditional India.)

Meditation on this Visuddhi or throat chakra with devotion to the Hindu Goddess of Learning, Saraswathi, is a potent method to awaken it. Many Hindu poets regularly worship this goddess with hymns and songs. It may be noted that in the Hindu pantheon of gods, Saraswathi is the divine consort of the Lord of Creation, the four-faced Brahma.)

The Ajna or eyebrow chakra is located between the eyebrows, inside the brain, close to the pineal gland. This is the place where Hindu ladies apply 'tilak' or a mark with red powder (kumkum) or with chandan. This is also the third eye or the wisdom eye of Lord Shiva, who is supposed to open this eye during his moments of anger or indignation. He used the fire from the third eye to destroy demons and to threaten those who opposed him in arguments.

The term 'Ajna' means *command*. This chakra helps to control the five sense organs and to regulate one's intuitive powers. Hence it is called 'Command chakra'. Many had misinterpreted this to mean 'command over others'. Yoga is not meant for command or control over others, but only to exercise restraint and command over one's own unruly senses. Some yogis have even threatened their gullible followers with their imaginary powers! (In the Upanishads, the senses are referred to as wild, unruly horses, to be reined by the mind – *Katha Upanishad*.)

This chakra can activate intuitive powers and extrasensory perception (ESP) to a great extent. Therefore, meditation on this chakra is done after one has advanced substantially, after at least one year of practise of meditation on other chakras. There are teachers who may suggest straightaway focusing on this chakra. This is a dangerous, misguided practice.

The author has read ridiculous procedures, apparently practised in Tibetan monasteries, such as the following: the master performs a ritual in which a small hole is drilled into the Ajna chakra location of the pupil, with a small tool, and a wooden sliver is pushed inside to press and activate the chakra. After that the wound is allowed to heal by applying some ointment. Such methods are unlikely to be practised but the authors write them mainly to mystify the methods for lay readers.

Incidentally, yoga and Kundalini literature are full of several imaginary, stupid and dangerous practices written by unscrupulous authors to create awe in the minds of readers.

During meditation on this chakra, ecstatic states may be experienced. One may feel extremely light or as if floating in air. One may observe a bright light, luminous objects, a blue star, a red ruby-like bright object and so on. These are merely projections of one's mind and should not be taken as any advanced state. The meditator should gently note them and ignore these as minor vistas on the way, like one sees several scenic views while travelling in a train. He should not discuss these small experiences with fellow students and compare notes or feel elated or puffed up with pride. For the most part, such experiences are of minor significance.

(This chakra is represented as a lotus with two petals. The two petals may signify nerves going to the left and right hemispheres of the brain.)

Meditation with eyes closed, or partially open, directed towards the centre of the eyebrows is the one most commonly practised. It requires considerable practice to meditate with the eyes open, though some yogis do this. Those who close their eyes must relax the body well before meditation so that they do not fall asleep during the session. In the initial stages, one can take a break after meditating for ten minutes to reduce the strain on the eyes.

Cleansing the Subconscious Mind

During the meditative process, the mind is cleansed of putrid thoughts, often relating to past, unpleasant events and guilty feelings. These thoughts are stored in the subconscious mind, just as we store old, discarded things in basement cellars or small attics. While our mind is calm during meditation, these thoughts may surface one by one. These are thoughts of guilt, fear, anguish, hatred and resentment, along with pleasant ones also. For many meditators, these early periods lead to mental pain and anguish; they may cry and even shout when these strong thoughts are felt deeply. You must, with patience, face them and learn to watch them with detachment. Tell yourself that this is your unpleasant past, to be forgiven or forgotten once and for all.

Many would say that it is easy to forgive someone, rather than forget what one has done or said to you. This process, through meditation, is an effective way of cleansing your subconscious mind of all old, dirty debris. This is referred to as *'Chitta Suddhi'* – purifying your mind. This step is essential for all meditators to pass through.

After about a week or two or sometimes a month, a person attains sufficient cleanliness of the mind, the meditation becomes peaceful and joy alone is experienced. As this process is gone through, one feels less tense after meditation and usually one's face shows less tension and fatigue. Most meditators report that their friends are able to notice a distinct change in their faces and often remark: "You look fresh and relaxed – what did you do?" ...You will see a change in your face and in your attitude towards day-to-day encounters. This feeling of relaxation is found to be more permanent than what you would experience after two weeks of vacation!

Meditation on the Ajna chakra is considered the most potent method of mental cleansing. After this, if you meditate on the heart chakra, your feelings of compassion and joy will be almost ecstatic.

Many, including the present author, have observed that after such mental cleansing, you will not get bad dreams at all. This is one of the easily observable effects. Furthermore, you will sleep deeply, almost like a little child!

Powers of Siddhi

Thaumaturgic powers, called siddhis, in Indian yoga, include several kinds of powers such as clairvoyance (hearing from a distant place), clairaudience (appearing in a distant place or being present in more than one place at the same time), premonition (getting to know what will happen in the near future), precognition (knowing an event beforehand) and extrasensory perception (ESP) of all kinds: The siddhis include the power to move objects at a distance (psychokinesis), feeling light like a feather, levitation, walking on water and several others that can be practised by a yogi. The *Yoga Sutras* mention eight major siddhis (*ashta maha siddhis*) and several minor ones.

When one practises deep meditation for a long time, one acquires some of these powers unsought. They are acquired without conscious effort on the part of meditators. Many yogis and saints would state that such powers come to them as a result of their pure love towards humanity. (Of these powers, precognition seems to be an easier power. Most people gain this power in times of crisis or emergencies, with reference to their dear ones.)

Some yogis consciously develop these powers, following Mantra yoga (chanting certain mantras), Kundalini yoga or Raja yoga practices as given in Patanjali's *Yoga Sutras*. There were several yogis with such abilities a few generations ago, especially in the first few decades of the 20th century, and one may find authentic newspaper accounts as well as photographs of their feats. It is difficult to find even a few yogis who can reliably demonstrate these powers today.

Some have demonstrated physiological effects like control of pulse and breathing in recent times. Maharshi Mahesh

Yogi and his followers have demonstrated levitation. Paramahansa Yogananda has mentioned this effect of Pranayama in his book *Autobiography of a Yogi.*

It is important to understand that any attempt to develop these powers is a waste of time and energy. Such practices are bound to drain both physical and mental energies. They are not to be practised for the purpose of demonstration, either to attract students or to make money. Yogis who do these things to create a mass following have spoiled the name of Yoga and Indian spiritual lore.

It is altogether a different matter when a great yogi or saint uses these powers to help a devotee in a specific instance. The example of Shirdi Sai Baba comes to mind. He never sought popularity or money, but had love for his disciples. He used his enormous siddhi powers to help them in times of crisis. Likewise, Edgar Cayce's readings were meant for public good.

Sahasrara Chakra

The Crown chakra or Sahasrara chakra is the centre with the thousand-petalled lotus and forms the ultimate place of liberation or mukti. The Kundalini raises to this chakra and merges with Purusha or the Lord there. This is a symbolic way of stating that the Jiva has merged with the Cosmic Force or Paramatman once and for all. According to many yogis, this is an irreversible process – once this union takes place, the person becomes liberated and lost to this world.

But there are divergent views. Such persons, of their own free will, may return to the mundane world or world consciousness and help humanity. If you believe in Jivan Mukti (liberation while in the human body) you may hold the view that such persons are Jivan Mukṭas living for some more years on earth. (This is the Advaitic view. Bhagwan Ramana Maharshi and Swami Nityananda were Jivan Muktas. There are or were many others who had claimed this state. Note that some philosophical systems do not accept the Jivan Mukti state at all – for instance Vishist Advaita of Sri Ramanuja and Dvaita of Sri Madhva Acharya). Jivan Muktas may live, sleep and eat like normal beings, but their mind is lodged in their Atman or Soul and remains unaffected or untainted.

Can one meditate on the crown chakra? This is the practical question we will address ourselves. The answer is 'yes' but after considerable practise of meditating on the Ajna chakra and heart chakra. Most saints and yogis would advise meditation only on the Ajna and heart chakras. Some prefer to meditate on the crown chakra, focusing on a point a few inches above one's head. The present author would suggest that one should practise meditation on the crown chakra only at the instance of an accomplished guru and not after reading a book of this kind or any self-help or yoga book. (Reiki practitioners do Reiki on that chakra following a different approach.)

The effects of activating the crown chakra have been written. The individual feels total equanimity with all creatures of the world (*samadrishti*) and feels consciousness of the entire universe (Cosmic Consciousness). He may have overwhelming love for humanity, without any fear whatsoever. He has transcended formal human life. (A great aura may be seen around the head of such a person.)

The present author believes that meditation on Ajna and heart chakra for at least ten years is required to attain the state before attempting meditation on the crown chakra. If they are well prepared, this process will be automatic and under the guidance of a guru who will reach such an advanced meditator. Nothing more can be said on this point at this stage.

> **Note:** *The awakening of Kundalini and the activation of chakras are possible purely by the devotional path or Bhakti Yoga. Some traditions use only mantras to activate chakras.*

Chakra Meditation – General Instructions

An important aspect of meditation on chakras should be discussed – the response of individuals to such practices. Almost all meditators at the initial stages are bound to face some discomfort or minor problems. These problems are mostly physical and mental discomfort due to the release of stresses and thoughts of past actions and their associated feelings.

Some may feel minor discomfort due to bodily pains and headaches. Some may experience sudden coolness or chills in certain parts of the body. It is common to experience sweating in certain parts – forehead, back of the neck and palms. These are areas that are usually highly stressed. Even when you are tense and worried and seriously thinking about a problem, you may sweat in these regions. These minor problems usually disappear after a week or two and need not frighten anyone. But if the problem persists due to certain chronic ailments, the meditator must stop the practice and consult a qualified physician.

Note that chakra meditation is a profound way of changing your mental and spiritual makeup. It is not easy to change one's mental structure in a matter of days. If you have crossed 30 years of age, you are already accustomed to certain thought patterns for the past (nearly) 11,000 days. Thousands of thoughts, with their associated actions and events, are lodged in your mind. These surface at various times, either in pleasant or unpleasant ways. You have to reconcile with all those thoughts in some way. During meditation some of the dominant thoughts will surface and demand your mind's attention. You are also likely to get several dreams that are events to clear your mind. According to Hindu philosophy, dreams help one to cleanse his or her mind and also remove the effect of bad karma or actions of the past.

It should therefore be understood that meditation on chakras is effective at a deeper level, but one should proceed slowly and should not expect results in a few days.

Therefore, claims made by some yogis and gurus that Kundalini can be awakened in a matter of days and taken to the Sahasrara and one can attain realisation by quick simplified methods are not only unreliable but also likely to mislead beginners on this path. Therefore, it is better to avoid such methods.

In the traditional Hindu Yogic practice, either by Raja Yoga or by Tantra, the meditator is given a lot of practise in chanting (*japa*), worship (*upasana*) and scriptural studies (*sravana*) by a teacher with strict discipline and a daily routine. These are required to prepare the mind to face the cleansing process during meditation.

In Vedantic tradition, one follows a three-step procedure: '*Sravana*' (hearing the doctrines and scriptures from a master), '*Manana*' (reflection and introspection of what has been learnt), and '*Nidhidhyasana*' (meditation on doctrines, concepts and practice). The importance of a guru to guide and to monitor, particularly in a quiet ashram (hermitage) cannot be underestimated.

A meditator may reach a stage when he sees no real progress or feels dejected during this practice. This is sometimes called 'spiritual dryness'. The monotony of practice can lead to this, with very little formal recreation. Almost all meditators go through this period of dryness, a sort of plateau in the 'learning curve'. It is better to talk this over with a guru or senior teacher or friend. One method is to have a short break for a week or a month. In India, one undertakes a pilgrimage or visits another ashram to provide a change of scene and to gain fresh perspectives. One may undertake a deep scriptural study for a week (*saptaha*) to refresh one's mind.

Practice 12: Meditation on Chakra

- Sit in the meditative posture.
- Do breath-watch for five minutes.
- Visualise one of the chakras, say Muladhara, with a lotus with petals upward.

- ✦ Focus on the energy flowing into that chakra from the heart centre for a minute.
- ✦ Affirm that you have energised that chakra.
- ✦ Offer 'thanks' to the Almighty or guru or Ishata Devata for this meditation.
- ✦ Take deep breaths three or four times.
- ✦ Opening the eyes if closed, take half a glass of water or milk or lemon/orange juice.

(Some would meditate visualising a lamp at the concerned chakra location, instead of a flower or lotus.)

11. Visualisation Meditations

There are several meditation techniques under the category of visualisations. In both Indian and western traditions, such methods have been practised from ancient times. These methods can be part of concentration methods.

In recent times, visualisation methods have gained popularity as a means of fulfilling one's normal worldly desires and goals. One may also use these techniques to gain self-confidence and overcome fear and despondency. These techniques go beyond simple affirmations and 'positive thinking' approaches taught by motivational speakers.

We present two simple techniques:

Practice 13: Creative Visualisation

- Take a few deep breaths. Stretch your body, especially hands, feet and neck.
- Close your eyes gently.
- Note your breath for a few minutes.
- Visualise a blank screen in your mind's eye.
- Visualise a white, cloth screen (rectangular) stretched frame.
- Visualise your favourite scenic spot (beach, mountain top, valley, garden) in that frame.
- Visualise as many details as you can in that picture.
- Do this for 5 to 10 minutes (start with at least three minutes).

> **Note:** *This practice will give you a calm mind, inner joy and help reduce mental tension. It is like taking a mini-vacation for a few minutes!*

General Aspects

Creative visualisation practice assumes that you believe in a Supreme Force or Cosmic Energy or God, which enables you to fulfil your desires and dreams. This belief enables you to realise your inner potential. Note that no one can promise that you will have all your dreams fulfilled. But the visualisation helps you draw your inner energies with faith in the Cosmic Power. Indeed your inner powers are due to the Cosmic Power but not easily recognised as such.

Creative visualisation comes easy for little children. They believe in 'impossible' things. But as we grow older, the realities of life gradually lessen our imagination and faith in ourselves. Creative visualisation techniques help to activate legitimate imaginative faculties. The dormant potential in you is slowly released. For instance, if you have artistic or musical talents but never used them, you may receive suggestions to try them by simple means. You may receive suggestions to meet certain people or try certain approaches in realising your goals. These come to you from within your own mind – this is the power of creative visualisation.

Practice 14: Creative Meditation for Healing

1. First you reach a lower level of alpha waves in the brain, which means a meditative state. Relax your muscles and body parts.
2. Take a few deep breaths.
3. You may lie down flat on a hard mattress or on the floor. You should not be too tired or else you may fall asleep. Stay awake and alert. Keep your eyes closed or half closed.
4. Slowly count from ten to one: ten, nine, eight...

5. Visualise the body parts that need healing.
6. In your mind's eye see that part as completely healed and with you being able to use that part fully.
7. If it is an internal part like the intestines, say an affirmation: "I am healthy; my _______is completely healed and functions as it did when I was young."
8. Repeat the affirmation thrice.
9. Visualise using that part in physical activities or games.
10. Slowly tell yourself: "With the grace of God, I am perfectly healed." Repeat thrice.
11. Slowly count 1 to 10: one, two, three....
12. Open your eyes gently and take a sip of water.
13. Repeat this process at least thrice a day.

Practice of General Aspects

You can practise the following general visualisation at least twice a day: in the morning after arising and at night before going to bed.

Follow the steps given in the previous practice.

Repeat the following affirmation:

"I am a radiant being, filled with Love. The Lord who dwells in my heart is creating a great and purposeful life Here and Now."

Repeat the affirmation thrice.

Thanksgiving

At the end of each visualisation session, offer 'thanks' to your teacher, parents, guru or God or master for the session you had.

12. Buddhist Meditations

We have mentioned a few Buddhism-related meditations, commonly practised by their monks. The breath-watch and mantra meditations are common to both Hinduism and Buddhism.

Tibetan monks practise meditation using the mantra 'Om Mani Padme Ham' (Om, the Jewel in the Lotus), focusing on the navel or Manipura chakra. This meditation is likely to bring creativity and prosperity to the practitioner. This has been discussed earlier.

In this chapter, we describe a few simple meditations to promote awareness, the presence of NOW and, above all, charity and compassion towards all. In fact, these aspects are the core of the teachings of Gautama the Buddha. (**Note:** *Gautama was his name after taking sannyas; his original name was Siddhartha; the Buddha means* 'the awakened'.)

These meditation techniques have been handed down through the generations from Vedic times, but mainly redefined by Buddhist monks. Though these methods were practised in India, China, Japan and Tibet, as the religion of Buddhism spread after 6th century BC, they were preserved better in isolated Tibetan monasteries. Therefore, they are often referred to as Tibetan Buddhist meditations' of Vajrayana (the diamond path) tradition. The traditions of Theravada (the way of the Elders) Buddhism in Ceylon have similar techniques. The Theravada tradition is also included in Vipassana or insight meditation.

This class of methods refers to constant awareness of oneself or one's own thoughts. We will discuss, in particular, the Samatha meditations, the four abodes of the Buddha, namely:

- Loving kindness
- Compassion
- Joy in the joy of others
- Equanimity

This meditation can be done alone or in pairs. Two persons sit opposite each other and look into each other's eyes... You visualise or imagine immense resources of intelligence, endurance, joy and wisdom behind those eyes.

From Joy we have come, in Joy we live and have our being, and
In that sacred Joy we will one day melt again.

—Taittriya Upanishad (3-6-1)

Practice 15: Joy Meditation

1. You let the feeling develop that the other person be free of pain and sorrow, failure and losses, grief and disappointments. You let the feeling develop of healing of resentments and mental hurts. (This is the aspect of 'healing meditation'.)
2. As you look into the eyes of the other person, let yourself be aware of your desire that this person be free from hatred and greed. You are now experiencing 'Loving Meditation'.
3. As you look into the other person's eyes, become aware about how ready you might be to work together for some common cause or public good, trusting each other, acting boldly with 'Joy in each other's Joy meditation'.
4. As you look into each others' eyes, open your consciousness to the deep web of relationships that underlie all experiences, with your knowledge – from what you are, from your being – feel the great peace;

out of that great peace, we can venture into many things, with trust, we act. This is the fourth 'Equanimity' meditation.

Buddhist literature says these meditations change the present moment with beauty and discovery; it opens us to the *sacredness of the moment.*

Husband-wife pairs can practise this meditation.

This meditation can be extended to non-humans also; the other being in the meditation can be an animal, a tree or a plant. *It is based on the firm conviction that all life is interconnected.*

The Lotus Meditation

There is an anecdote in the life of Gautama Buddha. Once he held a discourse in Benaras (Varanasi). He took his seat on the dais, adjusted his robes and looked at his followers. With compassionate eyes, he took a single lotus flower and held it high in his hand. He moved his hand from left to right, front and back, so that all could see the flower. Then he gently brought the flower close to his chest and held it there. The followers were eagerly expecting the Buddha to open his mouth and deliver a discourse. He kept silent. We are told that, out of the thousands who had gathered there, only a few understood the meaning of the meditation he preached by holding the flower.

Among flowers, the lotus occupies a special place in Hindu mythology. The lotus is a flower that grows in muddy waters. The mud represents our mundane life or samsara with joys and sorrows, with love-hate relationships. The lotus stalk rises above muddy waters, like our mind lifted out of such dispositions seeking divine light. Lotus leaves are not wetted by water. Our mind remains aloof from love and hatred. The flower blossoms when the sun shines. This is likened to the opening of our heart when knowledge or enlightenment dawns on us.

Practice 16: Lotus Meditation

1. Get a fresh lotus or any other flower (not a plastic one!).
2. Hold it at arms length and study its features.
3. Mentally affirm that the flower represents purity in thought, word and deed.
4. Slowly bring the flower close to your chest, all the time focusing your eyes on the flower.
5. Gently close the eyes and assume that the flower is inside your chest or in the heart centre.
6. Retain the image of the flower and assume that the flower slowly blossoms in full.
7. Hold this image for two to three minutes.
8. Make an affirmation: "With God's grace, I am a pure and radiant being." Repeat this affirmation thrice.
9. Gently open your eyes and leave the flower at the altar.

13. Benefits of Meditation

We shall discuss the benefits of meditation in terms of their effects on the body, mind and spirit.

Physiological Effects

Numerous studies conducted by the institutions of Transcendental Meditation of Maharishi Mahesh Yogi and of Swami Rama (the Himalayan International Institute) have demonstrated mainly physiological effects. These are reduction in blood pressure, pulse rate, breathing rate, and basal metabolic rate (BSR) among others. The alpha waves in the brain also decrease in amplitude. The pulse rate may be lowered and the pulse can be stopped for a few moments. It should be noted that these effects are seen at the time of meditation. The doctors investigate by attaching probes on meditators and record the responses during the specific practices.

(Here is an account published in *The Hindu* newspaper of 30 March 1936: "An interesting lecture on the subject 'Super Art of Living' was given by Swami Yogananda (later Paramahansa Yogananda) at the Gokhale Hall in Madras (now Chennai) on the 28 March 1936... At the end of his lecture, Swami Yogananda gave a demonstration of his ability to control at will his pulse rate. Doctors present found that as he went into deep meditation his pulse rate came down to only 16 beats per minute. Later, the Swami said that in ideal conditions he could, in fact, bring down that rate to zero by yogic withdrawal.")

What will be the permanent effects seen even after the meditation session? One can certainly notice reduced activity for an hour or two after the meditation. The long term or sustained effect of reduced blood pressure has been demonstrated. But several studies show that over a period of time, the blood pressure (both systolic and diastolic) reach low or normal levels, though the results may vary widely from person to person.

There are more tangible benefits. For instance, reduced muscular tension, whereby a greater feeling of well-being is felt by the practitioner. Meditators feel less tension in the body. Longstanding cases of headaches and migraine, neck pain and pain in the lower back may be relieved after a short period of practice.

Improved breathing leads to strength and vitality. Several meditators have felt relief from asthma and allergic lung problems, but no general claims can be made or substantiated due to wide variations in responses of individuals.

Note: *Some meditators develop headaches and neck pains due to release of stresses in the first week or two. If the pain does not subside later, one should consult a qualified physician.*

Many meditators and yogis observe marked changes about their person in a few months. For instance, the voice may become less harsh and very melodious. The harshness in the face may disappear. A gentle, pleasant face is easily attained. Some have reported the blackening of grey hair, with a lustrous shine. Again, results would vary and the author cannot make any promise on these aspects! Longstanding meditators, yogis and monks display an angelic countenance. This result will be seen only if the meditator or yogi is also strict about his/her diet and avoids spicy and pungent foods, and takes a very restricted quantity of food too. In ancient India, it was common practice among yogis/monks to take only one meal a day!

Most meditators develop eyes that are full of compassion and grace. It is difficult to describe such eyes in words. Only by seeing such accomplished yogis or meditators can one feel the penetrating power of their eyes. The author has had the rare fortune of seeing a few sadhus whose face and eyes he cannot forget.

Benefits for the Mind

Since meditation is largely a practice of mind control, benefits for the mind are immense, substantial and largely permanent. Firstly, the meditator develops intense concentration over a select topic or work. This has positive effects in one's day-to-day work and official or business career. The mind does not jump from one topic to another without control. Often a meditator acquires the ability to complete one task fully or to a satisfactory level before moving onto another. This ability is highly useful in our competitive world, when several distractions occur almost every minute. This ability in itself makes the meditator more focused and successful in his daily work and in his career.

Secondly, the meditator is not perturbed easily. He becomes a better listener. He calmly listens and takes in the information and is able to judge or make decisions with full awareness. This effect is documented only through anecdotes and no hard scientific research is available.

Thirdly, with calmness of mind, a meditator may develop phenomenal memory. This is due to fewer mental distractions. An experienced meditator can focus on a job even amidst noise and pestering distractions. Here again, specific studies are found wanting to 'prove' these effects.

Many meditators become more composed, less fidgety and less angry. Anger and resentment towards others will gradually disappear. One is able to forgive others easily. Here again, results may vary from person to person.

Spiritual Benefits

Meditation is essentially a spiritual practice or *sadhana*. The spiritual path is extremely difficult and is compared to walking along a razor's edge, according to the *Katha Upanishad*. Most of us follow, either consciously or unconsciously, the path of devotion or bhakti in the form of devotion to a God, guru or preceptor or some ideal. The path of devotion and worship (*upasana*) is considered easier, while the path of *gyana* and meditation is considered a difficult one. But such clear distinction of the two paths of bhakti and gyana is difficult to make for an individual. The two paths crisscross or merge at many moments in the life of a *sadhak* or practitioner. Therefore, Hindu tradition and other traditions have always combined prayer and meditation as a regular practice. In India, *japa* or chanting the Lord's name or a mantra is always recommended before one embarks on serious meditation practice. Some consider japa and meditation as two sides of the same coin.

Japa, selfless work (*karma yoga*) and meditation are, for the most part, steps to purify our mind from bad thoughts and feelings (*chitta suddhi*). When this is done effectively, the path towards spiritual goals becomes easier. This step can be compared to the civil engineer's task of clearing the land of weeds, boulders and stones, and levelling the ground before asphalt, tar or cement is spread on the road. Once the land is cleared, how easy it is to lay the road! Or consider a gardener who has to clear the soil of weeds and stones before planting flower saplings.

At the higher level, the spiritual benefit of meditation is, therefore, to understand and to merge with the Divine, conceived either as God with form (*Saguna Brahman*) or without name or form (*Nirguna Brahman*). The samadhi state is reached during moments of meditation. For many, this experience would be an extremely short period, say a few minutes. Even these short moments serve as intimations of the Blissful state (referred to as *Sarvikalpa Samadhi*) when one is aware of his/her consciousness. The memory of this experience remains forever, and the person is turned towards the godly, blissful path. Only a few persons attain the next higher state of *Nirvikalpa Samadhi* – when the individual consciousness or I-ness does not exist.

(We know from spiritual history that for saints like Ramakrishna Paramahansa, the state of *Nirvikalpa Samadhi* was a matter of daily experience, often extending to an hour or more. Sages like Bhagwan Ramana Maharshi remained always conscious of the Self, a state referred to as *Sahaja Samadhi.*)

Any meditation practice, however simple it may appear, is a step towards such superconscious experience. One need not be discouraged that such experiences are rare and reserved only for a few whom the Divine Being chooses or who can receive the Grace of God. *With faith in the Supreme Being or guru to lead us, we must keep trying.* No one can say when one would reach such an exalted state. If we are sincere, mentally pure and working towards the welfare of all, we are bound to receive proper guidance and help from the Supreme Being or Self. Meditation makes us fit to receive such grace or guidance or direction. It is said in the scriptures that if we walk towards God, He runs towards us.

Note: *One would not consider the attainment of siddhis or thaumaturgic powers or extrasensory perception (ESP) or the ability to predict the future as spiritual benefits of a high order. These powers are acquired unsought and may be used for the benefit of mankind – as Edgar Cayce and other clairvoyants did. If one works towards these powers and uses it to make money or hoodwink others, it would be a major disaster for the individual. The person will sooner or later face painful consequences and have a miserable end. The present author is aware of many such instances that cannot be mentioned here.*

14. Frequently Asked Questions (FAQs)

1. Is meditation easy to practise?

Yes. Meditation can be practised by people of all ages easily, if one follows step-by-step procedures. One should start with simple types of meditation.

2. How is meditation different from prayer?

In prayer, you seek help or guidance for a specific problem or for general good from the Almighty or the Supreme Force or God. You supplicate to the Lord with fervent appeal. You express in words what you seek.

In meditation, one quietens one's mind and tries to go within the mind and reduce thoughts. One seeks awareness of one's consciousness – to seek understanding of one's core 'Being'. In simple terms, one tries to forget the external world, but remains aware of his/her being. The outer world is forgotten at least for some time. One can start with prayer and later enter into a meditative state during the session.

3. Some say that meditation can lead to mental derangement. Is this true?

Meditation is a safe practice and will not lead to mental derangement. But certain yogic practices or Pranayama, if done wrongly, can be dangerous and could lead to mental derangement. They should be practised only under the guidance of a competent teacher. (We present only simple forms of breath control and do not recommend procedures like *bastrika* (bellow) type Pranayamas.)

4. Is meditation and surrendering to the Lord as in Bhakti Yoga (Yoga of Devotion) the same?

Meditation is a process in Gyana Yoga. This can lead to surrender to the Lord in later stages. At advanced levels, there is no difference between Bhakti and Gyana paths. A beginner can practise both the Bhakti marg and meditation at the same time.

5. What is Japa? What is meditation? How are they different?

In Hindu tradition, both japa and meditation are suggested as two steps towards spiritual growth. *Japa* is chanting the Lord's name (*nama japa*) or some mantra (*mantra japa*) given by a teacher or guru. Mere repetition of a name or mantra is sufficient to control one's wavering mind and focus on the desired God. But the process is considered very slow and may require several months or years of practice. Many sects, especially those of bhakti cult, suggest only nama japa, for instance, the followers of Chaitanya Mahaprabhu.

Meditation involves controlling the mind and reducing thought waves through watching the mind or breath or concentration exercises. The aim of meditation is to reach a state of awareness, or inner 'Being'.

According to Hindu tradition, japa and meditation are complementary techniques.

6. Some teachers advise complete detachment from worldly activities along with meditation. Will meditation lead to running away from home or taking sannyas (renunciation as a mendicant/monk)?

Meditation, as discussed in this book, is meant for householders and those who live an active worldly life. Meditation techniques as such do not lead to renunciation or detachment from worldly life. But if one chooses to become a sannyasi or monk, and then starts practising meditation as a preparatory step, it is a different matter.

7. Is it possible to acquire siddhis or psychic powers through meditation? If so, is it desirable to seek such powers?

Siddhis are special powers and yogic literature mentions eight major siddhis called *Ashta Maha Siddhis*. Some yogis and meditators do reach a level of attaining these siddhis. But siddhis should never be sought as a matter of course or as one's goal. The siddhis are considered distractions from higher spiritual pursuits. Some 'siddha purushas' or yogis may use these powers to help their disciples or the world at large. The siddhis, if attained, should never be used for harmful purposes. Then the downfall of the yogi will be great, leading to total ruin of his mind and body.

Psychic powers, such as precognition, clairvoyance, clairaudience, predicting the future and so on are more common among meditators and yogis. These are attained mainly due to calmness of the mind of the meditator. If external electrical noise is reduced, even a small radio with a short antenna can pick up distant, weak radio stations. Likewise, a calm mind can reach many thought patterns and records of events in the cosmic diary. Here again, a meditator should not talk about or vainly display his psychic powers. *One should not seek psychic powers and, if received as a by-product of meditation, should use the powers only for the good of others.*

8. Is it possible to materialise objects through meditation?

Some yogis/gurus claim to materialise objects such as sacred ash (*vibhuti*) or metal trinkets through spiritual powers. This is certainly not possible through meditation. If they do such materialisation through the practice of certain mantras, as claimed by some, the present author cannot substantiate such claims.

Meditation is meant for inner purification and control of mind and is not meant for creating objects of the physical world to attract or hoodwink others.

9. Can I achieve a higher degree of mental peace or 'shanti' through meditation?

The answer is a definite YES. In fact, a major aim of meditation is to achieve mental quiet, mental poise (balance), mental peace and tranquillity. The results are permanent; one attains the peaceful state for a long, long time, if one continues to meditate. For most persons, mental peace may be reached after a few weeks or a few months of practice. Those who have faced painful, traumatic experiences or have deep guilty feelings may require a longer time. The progress seen even after a few weeks will convince one about the efficacy of meditation. The mental peace is followed by a well-spring of inner joy to meditators.

10. Can meditation result in weakening of the body? Or will it lead to robust health?

As far as the author knows, almost all meditators have experienced robust health. Most common ailments such as cold, sore throat and headaches rarely occur to a meditator. Here again the results could vary depending on the past state of health, age, incidence of chronic illnesses and the duration of meditational practice. Sometimes a year of practice may be required before one attains a state of robust health. Meditation may be combined with Hatha Yoga, which is devoted to physical aspects.

11. Will meditation affect sexual passion?

Meditation helps to achieve normal levels of sexual passion or energies commensurate with your age and general health. Meditation will not eliminate sexual passion unless one makes a special effort or *sankalpa* towards suppressing or negating such passion. (Great yogis and monks learn to sublimate their sexual energies for spiritual progress. These aspects are not discussed in this book meant for general readers.)

12. What about visions and images one may see in meditation? Are they real? Do they convey any meaning to the meditator?

Visions and images seen during meditation are caused by projections from one's own mind. The meditator should not attach much importance: one may see blinding light or red gemstones or a golden moon and so on. They are as real as the images seen in a dream. If the images persist for several days, one can analyse and learn some message from the scenes.

Some would claim that angels and spiritual masters appear and convey messages through meditational sessions. They often appear in one's dream state when the mind is partially functioning and the senses are switched off. The meditational state does not support such visions. If one goes into a trance without one's control or awareness, that is a different state altogether and does not form part of conscious meditation.

13. Can meditation lead to healing of bodily illnesses? How does healing occur?

One should understand that there is a major difference between healing and curing. Curing is by an external agency – through drugs or surgical intervention. Healing is an internal process – your own immunity is increased and healing occurs. Through meditation, one increases one's own power of healing – by reducing physical and mental tensions, by improving mental functioning and above all, by reducing fear, nervousness and by auto-suggestion. Healers help to direct cosmic energy towards patients. (Some may practice Reiki or pranic healing along with meditation.)

14. Can meditation be effectively learnt through books, that is, without a teacher or living guru?

This is one of the most frequently asked questions. Meditation techniques can certainly be learnt from books. Hence this book!

Certain esoteric and complicated/hazardous techniques need a personal teacher or a guru. Alas, it is difficult to find teachers and gurus of high calibre and spotless character. In this field, as in many others, one finds many charlatans and bogus gurus who are interested in wealth and power. Therefore, it is safe to learn from books – at least the simpler techniques.

A personal teacher or guru is helpful in solving problems or sorting out difficulties during practice. But the other alternative of group practice in a large hall is hardly effective.

For higher levels of meditation or spiritual practice, Hindu scriptures assure that when a seeker is ready, a guru will be sent by Providence!

> **Note:** *It is important for a beginner seeking a guru to enquire about the guru from several sources and also to examine the behaviour pattern of the guru before joining or being brainwashed by the guru's disciples.*

Glossary of Sanskrit Terms

Anubhava	:	Experience, usually spiritual or mystic experience
Ashram	:	Literally, abode of saints, sages or teachers; also, the stage in life – the four ashramas denoting brahmacharya (student), grahasta (householder), vanaprasta (recluse) and sannyas (renunciant)
Bhakti Yoga	:	Path of devotion
Chakra	:	Literally, *wheel*; denotes nerve centres or nerve nodes
Gyana Yoga	:	Path of knowledge or self-enquiry
Hatha Yoga	:	Yoga of physical aspects
Manana	:	Reflection or introspection (of scriptures)
Mouna	:	Silence (of speech and thoughts)
Mudra	:	Gestures of hands, as in yogic postures and classical dance
Nidhidhyasana	:	Continuous or persistent meditation
Nirguna	:	Without attributes (without name and form)
Prarabda	:	Past acts, effect of past actions
Parampara	:	Lineage or tradition
Pratyahara	:	Withdrawal of senses

Sadhana	:	Practice, spiritual practice
Saguna	:	With attributes (with name and form)
Sat-sangha	:	Company of pious people
Sadhu sangha	:	Company of monks (monastery)
Samsara	:	Present actions, bondage of worldly life
Sandhya	:	Merging of time
Sravana	:	Study of scriptures, usually under a master in an ashram or gurukul
Upanishads	:	Part of Vedas, called Vedanta (philosophical parts of Vedas, *Gyana kanda*)
Upasana	:	Worship

Select Bibliography

1. Arthur Avalon – *Serpent Power* – Ganesh & Company, Chennai
2. Acharya Buddhavakita – *Living Legacy of the Buddha* – Buddha Vachana Trust, Bangalore
3. Andrew Weil – *Spontaneous Healing* – Sounds True Pub, NY
4. Andrew Weil – *Breathing: The Master Key to Self-healing* – Sounds True Pub, NY
5. Brother Lawrence – *Practice of the Presence of God* – Peter Pauper Press
6. Chogyam Trungpa – *Meditation in Action* – Shambala, Berkeley, USA
7. Davis, Roy Eugene – *Life Surrendered in God* – Centre for Spiritual Awareness, Lakemont, Georgia, 30552, USA
8. Daya Mata – *Only Love* – Yogoda Satsangha Society, Ranchi, 834 001, Jharkand, India/Self-realisation Fellowship, Los Angeles, USA
9. Daya Mata – *Finding the Joy Within You* – Yogoda Satsangha Society, Ranchi, 834 001, Jharkand, India/ Self-realisation Fellowship, Los Angeles, USA
10. Denning and Philips – *A Complete Guide to Creative Visualisation* – Llewellyn Press, St Paul, Minnesota, USA
11. Doriel Hall – *Healing with Meditation* – Gill & Macmillan Ltd, Dublin

12. Eckhart Tolle – *The Power of Now: A Guide to Spiritual Enlightenment* – New World Library, Los Angeles
13. Florence Scovell Shinn – *The Game of Life and How to Play It* – D B Taraporevala, Mumbai
14. Gawain, Shakti – *Creative Visualisation* – Bantam Books, NY
15. B K S Iyengar – *Light on Yoga* (Yoga Deepika) – Unwin Paperbacks, London
16. Le Shan, Lawrence – *How to Meditate?* – Little Brown Co Publishers, New York
17. Parthasarathy, A – *Vedanta Treatise* – The Vedanta Institute, Chennai
18. Ram Dass – *Journey of Awakening* – Bantam Books, NY
19. Swami Muktananda – *Where are you going?* – UBS Publishers, New Delhi
20. Swami Nirvedananda – *Hinduism at a Glance* – Ramakrishna Mission, Calcutta Students Home, Calcutta 700 056
21. Swami Shraddananda – *Seeing God Everywhere* – Advaita Ashrama, Calcutta 14
22. Swami Satprakashananada – *Meditation – Its Process and Practice* – Sri Ramakrishna Math – Chennai 4
23. Swami Sivananda Radha – *Hatha Yoga* – Timeless Books, Port Hill, ID
24. Swami Sivananda – *Meditation on OM* – Divine Life Society, Sivananda Nagar, Tehri-Garhwal, UP
25. Swami Prabhavananda – *The Yoga Aphorisms of Patanjali* – R K Math, Chennai 4
26. Swami Prabhavananda – *Spiritual Heritage of India* – R K Math, Chennai 4
27. Swami Virajeshwara – *Sadhana and Meditation* – Hamsa Ashramam, Anusoni, Dharmapuri Dt, Tamil Nadu, India 635113

28. Swami Vivekananda – *Raja Yoga* – Advaita Ashrama – Calcutta 14

29. Suzuki, Shunryu – *Zen Mind, Beginner's Mind* – Weatherhill, NY

30. Yogananda, Paramahansa – *Autobiography of a Yogi* – Self-realisation Fellowship, Los Angeles & YSS, Ranchi, 834001, Jharkand – India

31. K Vollman – *Journey Through Chakras* – Gateway Books, Bath, UK

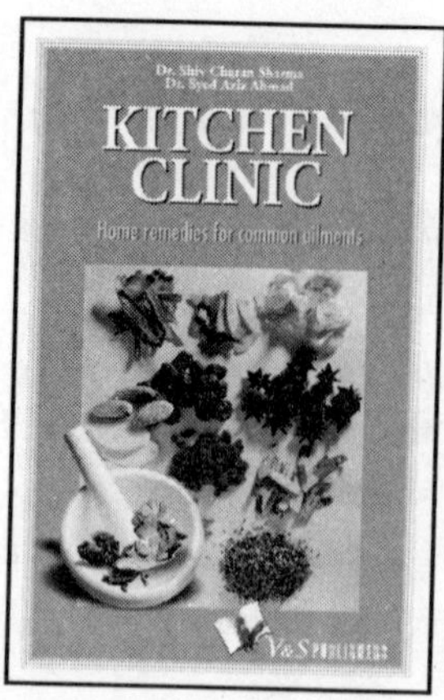

Kitchen Clinic
Home Remedies for Common Ailments

Home remedies and treatment of diseases by domestic plants have been prevalent since the time immemorial in India. The knowledge about the miraculous curing properties of plants is limited to certain people and is passed from one generation to another.

In the present book, the authors describe medicinal uses of 59 plants, which are used in daily life in the kitchen of Indian homes. Botanical names, vernacular names, identification, distribution and medicinal uses of each plant have been given. The book will serve as a guide of home remedies as practiced by our grandmothers, in the middle of night or at odd hours when drug stores are closed. This book gives some alternate ways of controlling earaches, insomnia, minor burns, coughs, eczema, sore throats etc.

Demy Size • Pages: 150

Dr. Ch. Murali Manohar
Ayurveda for All
Effective Ayurvedic self-cure for common and chronic ailments
Symptoms and Causes
Prevention and Treatment
Herbal Therapies & Nature Cure
Nutrition & Diet
V&S PUBLISHERS

Ayurveda for All

Recent years have seen a tremendous progress in the knowledge and practice of traditional Ayurvedic medicine, not only in India, but the world over.

Once treated with disdain, the exciting discoveries being pioneered by leading research scientists are proving that Ayurveda with its emphasis on health as well as disease is probably the world's most holistic health system.

As allopathic drugs extract a heavy toll in costs and side-effects, more medical many and more people worldwide are turning to complementary medical systems like Ayurveda, Homeopathy, Reiki, Acupressure and many others.

Big Size • Pages: 220

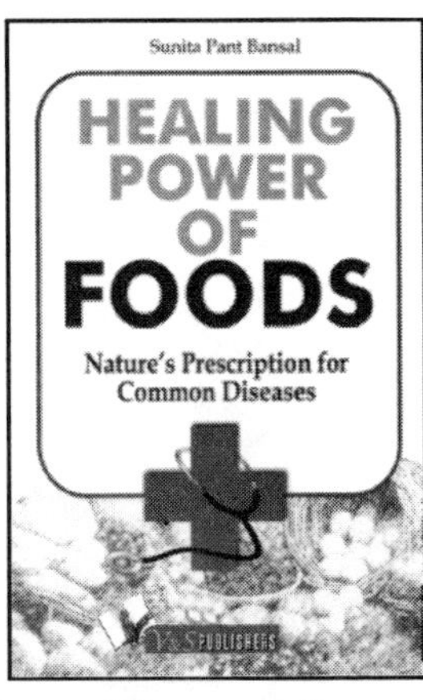

Healing Power of Foods

Hippocrates, the father of medicine, recognized that the medical therapy must be consistent with the nature and design of the human body.

He believed that the effective health care could not be separated from nutrition. He strongly recommended prevention of disease through balanced diet with a moderate and sensible lifestyle.

Hippocrates wrote, `Natural forces within us are the true healers of disease... Everything in excess is opposed to nature... To do nothing is sometimes a good remedy.` His philosophy was very much akin to the holistic health perspective of today.

The various foods in this book provide not only nutrition to our body, but prove to be medicinal too.

Demy Size • Pages: 130

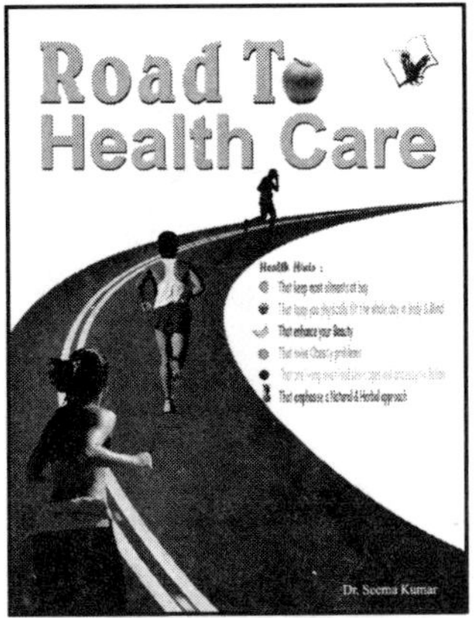

Road to Health Care

With ever-rising ground, water and atmospheric pollution, every other day one hears the name of a new disease. Ever since man began drifting away from Nature, he is falling into the trap of a materialistic lifestyle that has desensitised him. Today, we breathe air thick with exhaust fumes, eat processed junk food that has no nutritive value, drink toxic carbonated beverages and lead sedentary lives. All of this ensures that we are plagued with different kinds of problems at regular intervals. With natural preventive measures that emphasise diet, exercise and herbal remedies, there are no fears of obnoxious side effects.

Whatever be your problem – diabetes, blood pressure, asthma, acne, menopause, obesity, stomach ailments, premature ageing or general complaints – this book shows you a safe, natural and enjoyable means to overcome it. Most of the ingredients mentioned in the book are the kind available in home gardens or off the kitchen shelf. Once you have read this book from cover to cover, you need not rush to the doctor every now and then, but will be able to take care of your own and your family's health yourself.

Big Size • Pages: 176